POST-TRAUMATIC
SUCCESS

How to use traumatic events in your life to live your true purpose

DIANA BARDEN

Post Traumatic Success

How to use traumatic events in your life

to live your true purpose

First published in 2014 by

Panoma Press

48 St Vincent Drive, St Albans, Herts, AL1 5SJ, UK

info@panomapress.com

www.panomapress.com

Book layout by Charlotte Mouncey

Printed on acid-free paper from managed forests.

ISBN 978-1-909623-43-9

To Laurence and Lena
without whom none of this would
have meaning or purpose

Dear Sammy
Hope you enjoy reading
this!
Love Diane /x

WHAT PEOPLE ARE SAYING...

It's fantastic to have the spotlight shone on our vital support services and the many ways people can get involved and raise funds to help provide them. Breast Cancer Care is the only UK-wide support charity and with one in eight women developing breast cancer in their lifetime, there's never been such an urgent need for our support. The money raised through the donation from the sale of this book will ensure we can continue to provide our essential support services for free.

Samia al Qadhi, Chief Executive of Breast Cancer Care
www.breastcancercare.org.uk

This book gives a comprehensive guide on how to help yourself to success after a trauma, invaluable advice. I have known Diana for 20 years, a true and supportive friend, always sympathetic and very positive.

Jill Frances, Catering Manager at Skallywags
www.skallywagsnursery.co.uk

Diana is probably the best person I know to write this book as she is a very positive, driven person, with experiences many will never have. This book is well written and easily leads the reader to understand how they might make their life a little richer and also how to think success moving forward. An easy read for all, which will lead you to thinking about yourself with a new found anticipation!

Kevin Hard, Behavioural Consultant
www.kandocambridge.co.uk

I LOVE this book - I'm so pleased you're writing it and getting this message out there - it needs to be heard!

Caroline Reed O'Connor, owner of Bye Bye Pigsty
www.byebyepigsty.co.uk

Diana has a wealth of experience, both in life and in her career. Her ability to overcome adversity and turn that into a positive outcome, and her desire to help other people face adversity is testament to the power of this book. If you're feeling lost and need to find the reason why, I highly recommend reading Diana's book.

Guy Musgrave, Your Financial Architect
www.GuyMusgrave.com

How to some up such an ambitious and intelligent person in such a small space is what I am finding difficult. From the first day I met Diana her thirst for new knowledge and high expectation to succeed in life was just amazing to watch and see firsthand. In the years I have known Diana and her family I have been lucky enough to see her plans unfold. Although not always an easy journey, Diana would never been seen to give up or show weakness whilst following the plans for herself and her children. With confidence, professionalism and a love for what she does, Diana has proven to herself and everyone around her how successful you can be with faith, determination and a confident character that everybody can get on with. Diana has been a great role model in my life, inspiring me to study and pursue careers that I once thought were impossible. Diana is a fantastic mother, inspirational business women and friend.

Antonia Zirker, Director Zirker Gifts
www.facebook.com/ZirkerGifts

This book is a wonderful example of taking the worst possible difficulties that life can throw at you and turning them into a force for good. Diana's approach is both inspirational and practical. Highly recommended.

Ian Crocker – Absolute Learning
www.absolutelearning.co.uk

This book is a brilliant A-Z of what we can DO after we've been hit with a BIG unexpected trauma in our life - the bit where it really doesn't go according to our plan - it's about putting the 'right' ingredients into the Sausage Machine - this book is about Stepping Up when that negative voice in our head says "sit down" - it asks the question "what would you choose" A great book for all.

Richard Wilkins, UK Minister of Inspiration
www.theministryofinspiration.com

We all have traumatic events that affect us in different ways, and upon many levels during our lives. What's important is how we use those experiences to transform ourselves. Post-Traumatic Success is an honest and humorous account of using our experiences to develop ourselves and become who we want to be. A must-read for anyone feeling overwhelmed with life, from a truly inspiring woman.

Emma Hales, Owner of Press Any Key
emhales@icloud.com

ACKNOWLEDGEMENTS

No book is written solo, without immense help, input, feedback and support from other people. Some of those people know they are helping in the book's creation, others unwittingly provide material, anecdotes and even confidence boosts along the way. This book is no different.

I didn't know this at the start, but this book has been 20 years in the making. So many people have helped its creation in ways they could not imagine; if they only knew the impact they have had on my life, my health, my learning and the confidence I finally found to write this down. Aside from my family, who never fail to rally around when trauma strikes, I owe a huge debt of gratitude to the locum GP who had the intuition to worry about my breast lump more than I did back in late 1993, and who persuaded me to agree to a biopsy. Unfortunately I never discovered her name. I will be forever grateful to the medical team(s) who have picked me up and put me back together again, not just physically, when trauma has struck. James Bristol and Sue Kendall in particular have my undying gratitude.

My many mentors, teachers and coaches who have accompanied me on my learning journey in the Post-Traumatic Success years have contributed hugely to the insights and lessons contained in this book: Tony Robbins, Jamie Smart, Dan & Lucie Bradbury, Peter Thomson, Richard Wilkins, Topher Morrison and many, many others it would take me another whole book to list.

Thank you also to my trusted friends, Jill Frances and Emma & Stuart Hales and Caroline Reed O'Connor who kindly and generously gave me feedback on the first draft of this book. Your help was invaluable.

I have worked with many hundreds, if not thousands, of clients over the years, and the reason I love what I do is largely down to the opportunities they give me every day to learn – new ideas, new distinctions on things I thought I already knew, new ways of seeing the world. I thank every single one of my teachers who have given me more than they will ever realize.

I am immensely grateful to the professional team who packaged the ramblings of my mind into this book: Alison Baugh, my editor, Charlotte Mouncey, design and typesetting, and Emma Herbert for project managing the process. Finally, thank you to Mindy Gibbins Klein for not letting me off the hook when I first decided to write *Post-Traumatic Success*, and for never allowing my excuses to get in the way of the goal.

CONTENTS

INTRODUCTION

You have decided to pick up this book, so I guess something sparked your interest in the concept of Post-Traumatic Success. If you have lived through a traumatic event in your life, you may have gone through a period of confusion, wondering what it was all for, and perhaps even questioning why you had to go through this experience. No matter how long ago the traumatic event was, the chances are you went through, and perhaps still are going through, a range of emotions about the event itself.

Perhaps you have thought about what it meant, how you were supposed to deal with it and what life was trying to tell you. Did you blame yourself for the event? Did you look for the reasons why it happened to you, you of all people? Perhaps you believed before the traumatic event that such things only happened to other people.

I have been through similar thought processes and incessant questions myself. On New Year's Eve 1993 I was diagnosed with breast cancer at the age of 32. The diagnosis rocked the very foundations of my world. I was not ready for it, I was not prepared for it, and I had absolutely no references at all for how I was supposed to feel or how I was meant to conduct myself.

Just at the point where I began to think maybe I'd got away with it, nearly five years after my diagnosis, I was diagnosed with a malignant melanoma on September 16, 1998. In many ways the second diagnosis was worse; both were delivered appallingly, by doctors who I can only assume have never been given bad news, and have not been trained to give it.

The melanoma felt much more devious; there was no lump, no dramatic discovery in the shower, just a very innocuous-looking mole on my leg. I felt much more out of control, as I hadn't 'found' the offending collection of misbehaving cells myself. I felt somehow irresponsible and guilty – irresponsible that I had let this happen to me through years of unprotected sunbathing, guilty that *I* was putting my family through this trauma *again*, for the second time in five years. It felt as if I was somehow going overdrawn in that goodwill bank account of cancer sympathy and support. As I write this, the absurdity of that statement leaps off the page at me, and yet at the time I really believed it.

In 2003 my husband, the man who had stood by me through both lots of treatment, the man I thought I would grow old and sail into the sunset with, left me for an older woman. The jury's out on whether that's worse than being left for a younger model – I can't decide. At the time, I had two very young children still in diapers and a fledgling business in corporate training. I thought things were supposed to get easier once the cancers were behind me, and we had achieved our dream of having a family despite the years of harsh cancer treatments.

Those traumatic events were the beginning of my personal development journey.

These events have allowed me to learn things about myself I would not have learned otherwise, and could never have discovered without the events as triggers. How do you know, for example, how resilient you can be in a crisis if you never have a crisis to practice on? How would you ever find out just how resourceful you can become unless you find yourself standing on the edge of an abyss, believing you have nothing left?

These are the events that have led to *Post-Traumatic Success*. I have been traveling along my own Post-Traumatic Success path for the past 20 years, learning something new at every fork in the road, trying things out, making mistakes and trying again. I have learned how to become resourceful and resilient in the face of adversity, I have learned how to reprogram that internal voice that tries to shoot me down and make me feel small and somehow disapproved of, and most importantly, I've learned how to ask others for help, and not try to be Superwoman (okay, I'm still working on that one!).

This book is a further step on my Post-Traumatic Success journey. The name for the book has been sitting in my head for a long time. It seems the obvious description for those of us who want to make the traumatic events in our lives mean something.

There are some people, you and I both know them, who live their lives in Victimville – they seem to have such terrible dramas in their lives, they seem to be the unluckiest people on the planet, they never seem to quite get their lives together because just before they do, they are beset by another drama. These people believe things happen to them because they are genetically unlucky, picked on by the world at large in some great universal conspiracy, or because they are just bad people.

This book is not intended for these people. They are not ready to set out on their Post-Traumatic Success journey yet. I'll get to these people one day. For the moment I'd like to focus my attention on people like you: people who have come through something traumatic in their lives, and who believe they are meant to use the event for positive means. Everyone's Post-Traumatic Success dream will be different; for some it will be entirely altruistic and for the good of others, while for others it may be the courage to climb off the hamster wheel and go traveling, take up an extreme hobby they would never have dared do otherwise, start their own business or write a book. For me it's been all of these.

So I guess the reason you're reading this book now means you're ready to embark on your own Post-Traumatic Success journey for real. I congratulate you for that, and wish you all the luck and fun in the world. I believe wholeheartedly that whatever path your Post-Traumatic Success dream is meant to take, it will help you to give meaning to the traumatic event(s) in your life and will allow you to perceive it/them in a way that traumatizes less and comforts more.

I have been interviewed many times about my cancer journeys, through diagnosis, treatment and the subsequent years of follow-ups. One question I am always asked is what I would advise others who have been through similar. This is an impossible task, of course, since someone else's experience of the same traumatic event will be entirely different from mine.

One thing I have learned along the way is that your traumatic event is just that – an event, one of many events you will experience in your life. In and of itself, that event has no meaning. It does not mean you're a bad person or that you're inherently un-lucky – unless you choose to give it that meaning. The glass is not half full or half empty – it's a glass with liquid in it. Whether we choose to see it as half full or half empty is a direct result of the meaning *we choose to project on to it*.

You are not your trauma. I am not my cancer or my marital status. You are not your debt, your employ-ment status, your sexual orientation or any other label that society loves to give to categorize us. That is a part of you, a part of your journey so far on this plan-et. How *you* choose to use that label is *your* choice. Per-sonally I find labels rather itchy and irritating; I prefer to cut them out!

What if you were to view a traumatic event as but one act in the great masterpiece that is your life? If you were watching a play in the theater it would not make a lot of sense if one act were to be omit-ted because it's a bit unpleasant or uncomfortable. The other acts would not hang together and your enjoyment of the play would surely suffer. Trouble is, there is no blueprint, no rule book or operating manual for how to deal with traumatic events, how to incorporate them into the masterpiece so it hangs together and makes sense.

That is what I have tried to provide with this book. Some scenes in a masterpiece will always be more memorable than others as you look back over the whole play; some have more action sequences or dramatic effects, others have more memorable characters or are more shocking. Some scenes stand out because for some reason you feel more connection to them. My hope is that as you embark upon your Post-Traumatic Success journey by reading this book, you will find the right meaning in *all* the scenes that go to make up the masterpiece of your life.

Diana Barden

November 2013

CHAPTER 1

"You were sick,
but now you're well again,
and there's work to do."

Kurt Vonnegut, *Timequake*

Trauma? What Trauma?

*"Please come back in and close the door, Miss Whitehead,
I need to go through your histology results with you. I'm
afraid the biopsy shows the tumor in your breast is cancer-
ous, so you're going to need further treatment."*

That was New Year's Eve 1993.

The reason the surgeon asked me to come back into
his consulting room was I had assumed, wrongly as it
transpired, I was merely having the stitches removed
following the biopsy a week earlier, and since that was
completed, I was free to go. I had already said good-
bye, wished him a Happy New Year, and was on my
way out the door. I stopped dead in my tracks, assuming I had misheard.

I was totally stunned by this news, as I expect most
people are when they receive a cancer diagnosis. In
my case, however, I was particularly taken aback because a week earlier the same consultant had stood

outside the recovery ward where I was coming round from the anesthetic, and assured my worried mum that the tumor 'looked benign'. Now, a week later, and on New Year's Eve of all days, I was being given what to me sounded like a death sentence, and this at the tender age of 32 years, seven months and four days.

All sorts of thoughts were rushing around in my head, randomly crashing into each other in their desperation to be heard and processed by the analytical part of my brain:

How am I going to break the terrible news to mum?

This has to be a mistake, I'm only 32 for God's sake, 32-year-olds don't get breast cancer.

I've never had the opportunity to have children.

Thank God I don't have any children, who would look after them if I died now?

I've just paid £8,500 to study for my MBA, what a waste of money if I'm going to be dead before I graduate.

I'll get a second opinion, this doctor doesn't know what he's talking about.

Thank God Dad isn't alive, he had a pathological fear of the Big C, the news would have killed him. (Yes, that really was one of the thoughts careering around in my head)

The concept of Post-Traumatic Success has been incubating inside me for a number of months, maybe even years now. You see, I've met many hundreds of people over the last 19-plus years who are survivors of all sorts of traumas: life-threatening or life-changing illness, divorce, bereavement, rape, redundancy, infertility, violence, early onset menopause... the list is endless. And for many of these people there is something fundamental about the trauma they have experienced and survived: that is, the trauma has changed them. It has changed them in the same way as breaking an egg changes the egg; once poached or fried, the egg will never fit back into the shell.

The trauma changes its 'victim' physically in some cases, just like the egg, but even more than that, it changes its victim mentally, emotionally and psychologically in ways that are more profound than just that which is seen.

The removal of a breast or a limb, for example, will leave a person's body looking different. Modern prosthetics can go a long way toward recreating the original shape and enabling a level of activity through artificial limbs; however, the mental and emotional scars can remain in place long after everyone has stopped asking you how you are. They can last a lifetime if left to fester in secret. And that's just it; often they do remain secret for months or even years – secret from our friends and family,

and more destructively, secret from ourselves.

I remember this being the case for me; a few days after my diagnosis, once I'd had a chance to let the news sink in, I started telling a few close friends and family that I had breast cancer. Of course people were very sympathetic, supportive and keen to help in any way they could. People brought cards, flowers, heartfelt wishes, and I really appreciated those.

I appreciated them all the more as I had just uprooted my life to live in a country that had become foreign to me over the 10 years I had been living abroad. In 1993 Facebook was still 11 years away, so the wishes came personally, by phone and by letter. As the plan for my treatment came together, friends and family stepped forward to drive me to hospital for appointments, to sit with me at home, to take my mind off the cancer for a while. I was grateful as it also took some of the pressure away from my mum.

When Normal is No Longer Normal

There comes a time in anyone's trauma, however, when those around you just want things to go back to 'normal'. They want to be your friend not your care-giver, they want to be able to have a laugh with you, without treading on eggshells and worrying that laughing means not showing sufficient respect for your trauma. I know, I've been on both the care-receiver and the care-giver side of the equation. If you've been through your own trauma, you'll know exactly how that felt for you to be the care-receiver; it can be debilitating, disempowering and destabilizing, yet life on the care-giver side can also become wearing, hard work, energy-sapping and uncertain. From a purely practical point of view you might need to arrange your own life around your friend or relative's hospital appointments, counseling or need for short notice tea-and-sympathy dates. In the longer term, decisions may need to be made for longer term changes in lifestyle for the 'traumatized' person.

From a psychological-emotional point of view, the balance has shifted. As friends, you might have had a fairly balanced relationship, where each looked to the other for specific things: approval, confidence, companionship, knowledge or fashion tips, for example. In the care-giver/care-receiver relationship this balance tips; what may have felt quite equal before is no longer equal. One party needs, the other provides. Now, I realize it may not be quite as stark as this, nevertheless there is likely to be a shift in behavior, in expectations, even in the language you use with each other. You might find you check yourself before speaking so as not to use a word or phrase that could cause upset or be construed as insensitive.

What's So Great About Normal Anyway?

I had a fairly unremarkable childhood in many ways, and yet there were enough aspects of it which made me feel different – different from other children at school, different from my family and certainly different from what was expected of me on many occasions. Different does not necessarily mean bad; for a child, however, it can mean the difference between being in the 'in-crowd' looking out or feeling like the outsider with your nose pressed against the window, imagining what it must be like to be 'in'.

Not that anything terrible happened to me – I wasn't bullied, I didn't go through any life-threatening situations (those came later) and I didn't run away and join a sect. And yet somehow I always felt different.

Being born in Birkenhead on the Wirral has always allowed me to build a connection with my friends, colleagues and clients from the north of England, although if you have ever heard me speak, you'll know I certainly don't sound like a Northerner at all! We moved when I was three months old to California, the other half of my heritage, and lived there for the first year of my life. In a similar vein, my Californian genes allow me to join in US-focused banter with the caveat that I'm allowed to be cynical – after all, I hold a blue passport. I also don't sound American to those who know me.

For part of my early childhood we lived on a dairy farm while my dad lived out his dream of working with animals. We had around 60 dairy cows and many hundreds of battery hens. Before you judge, we're talking the mid-1960s, before the days where hens were politically organized and realized they could have a better life running around in the open.

I earned my first pocket money at the age of around four or five, grading eggs into four sizes: small, medium, standard and large. This was done by means of a very high-tech piece of equipment known as an egg grader. It was a piece of thick cardboard with four different-sized holes in it, so my job consisted of carefully placing each egg into the holes, holding it carefully to stop it dropping through, to find the snuggest fit, and placing it carefully into the appropriate cardboard tray. For this very responsible task I earned three pence a week. If only I had known then what I know now about the effects of compounding – I could have retired on the proceeds of my income as a four-year-old.

I returned to the land to earn a pretty good teenage income when I reached high school, and spent several summers picking strawberries, raspberries, plums and apples for a local farmer. On a good day I could earn a better hourly income than the 66 pence an hour I earned in my Saturday job on the till at Macmarket supermarket!

Trendsetter – Without Followers!

Back to the farm years; I think the first time I felt acutely aware of being different was when I started school. My first elementary school was Hollycombe Primary School in a hamlet called Milland on the Sussex/Hampshire border. This in itself was not unusual; however, what for me was the source of cringing embarrassment was the fact that the school was situated at the end of the corner field of our farm. While all the other children arrived at school by car (remember the old A40s and the Morris Minors with the goldfish indicators?) and wearing standard attire for the four-year-old of the day (pre-school uniform times), I was made to walk across the muddy field in very untrendy skinny jeans and rubber boots. Oh, the embarrassment of it! Who knew that combination would become the ultimate fashion statement for four-year-olds and adults alike a mere 50 years later? If only I'd known I wasn't different at all, just ahead of my time! That said, when my own daughter was four and went through the 'Rubber Boot Phase' – rubber boots with everything – I was traumatized all over again! How could any self-respecting four-year-old *choose* to wear rubber boots if they didn't have to?

My second memorable event happened at the same school two years later. Hollycombe was made up of two classes: Infants and Juniors. That meant when my brother started school, he came into my class, even though I was, of course, academically light years ahead! By this time our neighbors on the farm and I had neatly resolved the rubber boot dilemma; we would hide our boots in the hedge at the corner of the field and put on our indoor shoes to walk the last 100 yards or so to school in a boot-free manner. This allowed us to hold our heads high and repress our embarrassment to an indefinite time in the future where we (or at least I) would release the years of pent-up psychological trauma and rubber boot demons in a book!

My brother was a different kettle of fish altogether. Not understanding the gravity of the whole rubber boot situation, he insisted on keeping his boots on for the entire journey to school, and would not be moved on the issue. Grudgingly we allowed him to keep his boots on for the day! Now as if that weren't social impairment enough for a six-year-old, having a brother in tow who insisted on keeping his rubber boots on, to add insult to injury he had managed to break his arm a few weeks before starting school, and so had a plaster cast on his arm. Talk about psychological scarring (for a socially ambitious six-year-old)!

The situation came to a head at lunchtime on the first day, when the whole class was expected to file into the washroom to wash their hands before lunch. Everyone duly filed in and back out apart from my brother, who didn't reappear from the hand-washing task. The teacher was about to send someone in after him, when the bathroom door flew open, and he stood in the doorway, sobbing loudly. "Whatever is wrong?" asked the teacher, concerned he had somehow hurt his broken arm, or perhaps even the good one. "I've washed my good hand, but now I can't dry it because I can't hold the towel with the other hand!" he wailed.

It was at this point that I behaved in a way that with years of hindsight and personal development I'm not entirely proud of. However, in my defense, you're beginning to build a picture of my desire, indeed my basic human need, to feel 'normal'. The teacher asked who would be prepared to go and dry Brian's other hand. Now, I know what you're thinking: being the big sister, the responsibility to go and put him out of his rather embarrassingly noisy misery lay squarely with me. Well, that's easy for you to think; with respect, you weren't there, and you don't understand the toll that social pariah-hood had already taken on my fragile self-esteem, rocking up to school with a brother in rubber boots and a plaster cast!

Just Different

Fast forward a few years, and several schools; my feeling that I was different from others continued to be perpetuated with every house move, every school change, every new set of friends. When I was 10, we moved to the Midlands, the part of the country I still consider 'home' when I visit, even now. It seemed a million miles away from leafy Surrey; it looked different, the climate felt different, people even spoke differently!

The first year, which was my last year of elementary school, was spent trailing around high schools and being drilled for exams. I must have taken every past paper for the 11-plus exam, as well as learning every revision guide for the Common Entrance that was available in those heady pre-internet days. In the end I differentiated myself once again from my friends by passing both, and once again found myself alone in a new school, making yet more new friends a year later.

I feel no judgment, either positively or negatively, to the feeling of being different from the rest of the world; I accepted the feeling for what it was, and worked on the assumption it was 'normal' to feel like that. Being an extreme extrovert I always craved connection with others, and generally speaking, found it. Moving around from one school to the next meant that for most of my school years I didn't have a 'best friend' as the best friends were all taken by the time I arrived in a school. In retrospect this probably suited the extrovert need for an audience rather than a best friend.

Feeling different from my friends and family was not traumatic for me; the traumatic times came later in adulthood, when it could be argued I was big enough and tough enough to be able to deal with them. Although I did not know it at the time, the feeling different during my schooldays did prepare me in some small way for the huge difference one feels when hit with what objectively may be seen as a traumatic event.

Of course we all experience traumatic events differently and have our own ways of responding. Below is a list of the most common events that can be traumatic for the best of us. The list was compiled by Holmes and Rahe. In 1967 they examined the medical records of over 5,000 medical patients as a way to determine whether traumatic events might cause illnesses. Patients were asked to tally a list of 43 life events based on a relative score. These events are listed here in order of severity.

To measure the level of trauma according to the Holmes and Rahe Stress Scale, the number of 'Life Change Units' that apply to events in the past year of an individual's life are added and the final score will give a rough estimate of how the traumatic event can affect a person's health.

Sources of Trauma

Life Event	Man Value
Death of spouse	100
Divorce	73
Marital separation	65
Jail sentence	63
Death of close family member	63
Personal injury or illness	53
Marriage	50
Fired at work	47
Marital reconciliation	45
Retirement	45
Change in health of family member	44
Pregnancy	40
Sex difficulties	39
Gain a new family member	39
Business readjustment	39
Change in financial state	38
Death of close friend	37
Change to different line of work	36
Change in number of arguments with spouse	35
High mortgage	31
Foreclosure of mortgage or loan	30
Change in responsibilities at work	29
Son or daughter leaving home	29
Trouble with in-laws	29
Outstanding personal achievement	28
Spouse begins or stops work	26
Begin or end school	26
Change in living conditions	25
Revision of personal habits	24

Trouble with boss	23
Change in work hours or conditions	20
Change in residence	20
Change in schools	20
Change in recreation	19
Change in church activities	18
Change in social activities	18
Change in sleeping habits	16
Change in number of family get-togethers	15
Change in eating habits	15
Vacation	13
Christmas	12
Minor violations of the law	11

For anyone scoring more than 300 there is a major cause for concern. All life events within the past two years qualify.

This scale is adapted from Holmes and Rahe's Life Change Index.

Until I faced breast cancer in 1993, nothing in my life to date had really featured on this list. Yes, I had moved house and changed schools a few times, but none of those events was particularly traumatic. In fact, if anything they strengthened my natural resilience and gave me the inner core I came to rely on later, when I did experience traumatic events in my life.

I didn't know it at the time, but the changes I experienced in my early childhood provided essential lessons and stepping stones that were to serve me well later in my life. I have experienced a number of traumatic events as an adult, each of which on its own could have caused me to retreat into my shell and 'become' my trauma. With each traumatic event I have become stronger and more resilient, more able to face the next lesson as it was served up. I was able to see each lesson for what it was, take the learning from it, graduate and progress.

The Next Door Opens

The interesting thing for me over the years has been the way that I have experienced traumatic events in my life as leading to something positive. Not immediately, of course, but shortly after a traumatic event I have experienced something positive that would not have happened, or would not have happened to such an extreme, had it not been for the traumatic incident that preceded it.

In fact this realization is what has led to this book, indeed the whole concept of Post-Traumatic Success.

Let me explain. My breast cancer diagnosis came at the end of 1993, just at the end of the first semester of my MBA (Master's Degree in Business Administration). Now, I had started the course with some trepidation, I might tell you. I was one of 113 mature students, all of whom had been in the workforce for a number of years prior to their enrollment. Warwick Business School was a scary place; of 113 students on the course, there were 10 women, each one seemingly more professional, together and supremely more qualified to be there than me! The 103 men also seemed to have illustrious careers behind them; in fact the previous employers' names on everyone's resume read like a list of the FTSE100 index.

I felt anonymous, alone and very out of place in the first few weeks. I wasn't at all sure my experience in the working world matched up to or even came close to that of the lawyers, accountants and business managers in the room. I had been working for Bosch in Germany, safely cocooned in the bosom of the HR department, equally safe in the knowledge that my competence went unquestioned. After all, I was living and working entirely in a foreign language, and that earned me a certain kudos among my friends and colleagues.

During that first semester, in a time I often refer to as BC (Before Cancer), I met the man who was to become my husband and the father of my two children. I didn't know that at the start, of course. In fact my diagnosis served in many ways to speed up the start of our relationship. The second semester started the day I went into hospital to begin my treatment – January 11, 1994 to be precise. He came to visit me in hospital the day of my operation; I don't remember too much about that visit as I was still doped up to the eyeballs with anesthetic and morphine.

Whatever sight befell him, it seems it wasn't bad enough to scare him off as he visited every day I was in hospital, and continued to visit after I went home to recuperate. This was not as straightforward as it might sound – it was well over 100 miles round trip, and he made it during the precious time we all needed every evening to prepare for lectures and complete the relentless stream of reading, assignments, more reading and yet more reading.

He would relate what had happened during the day: who had fallen out with whom, who had asked a stupid question during a lecture, and always who had asked after me. I had only told one other girl on the course about my breast lump during the BC weeks on the course. I had been carrying the lump around with me for 18 months to that point, as doctors in Germany assured me it was benign. In fact the only reason I agreed to the biopsy was to appease the university doctor who looked visibly shaken when I told her of its existence. I had been happily convinced in Germany that it was a collection of friendly cells that were doing no one any harm.

So as far as I was aware, only two people out of the other 112 knew of my plight. Of course, the course administrators knew, as I had had to discuss my options for continuing my studies within 24 hours of being told it was cancer, while still coming to terms with the enormity of it myself. It transpired the lecturers had not been informed of the reason for my absence, so just at the precise moment I was going under the knife on January 11, the marketing lecturer decided to call out my name in a lecture hall of 112 students. When I didn't answer he made some rather crass assumptions (loudly, apparently) that the reason for my absence might have involved alcohol consumption the night before. In a valiant attempt to clear my tarnished reputation, my husband-to-be had to announce to the whole class that I was in hospital.

Any worry of anonymity, of not being up to the challenge, of being the weak link in a syndicate group that relied on each other for assessed coursework, all disappeared in that instant. I returned to the course exactly two weeks into the second semester to a rapturous welcome. As an extreme extrovert, even I was taken aback at the outpouring of love and connection.

And do you want to know the most interesting part? The number of my male co-students who came up and asked me about the lump, the diagnosis, the treatment, the emotions. I was amazed. I think alongside the genuine care for me, seeing someone their own age being diagnosed with an 'older woman's disease' really shocked them. I know for a fact that several of them who had cell phones (the size of house bricks in those early days) got them out and pleaded with their wives and girlfriends to check their breasts for lumps that night.

Over the next few years, my breast cancer opened all sorts of doors and engendered many, many conversations that would never otherwise have happened. I met people I would never have connected with in any other circumstances. I've discovered over the years there's a certain camaraderie among women who have been through a similar experience. I've also discovered that you'll find no group of people more raucous and free of taboos than a group of breast cancer survivors. Absolutely anything goes! Nothing, but nothing is out of bounds!

I met the woman who was at a grand charity auction, the first time she'd dared to wear a low-cut evening gown since her diagnosis, and, thinking she was pulling a handkerchief out of her bra, in fact flung her prosthesis into a complete stranger's beer glass! What about the woman who was groped on a crowded subway train and the groper managed to dislodge her prosthesis and somehow ended up with it in his hand! The next thing she saw was him out cold on the floor with the shock, still holding the offending boob!

An important milestone in my Post-Traumatic Success journey (although I didn't know it as such back then) was my successful application to join Breast Cancer Care as a peer support volunteer in November 1996. Here I've been privileged to enjoy opportunities, conversations, lessons and deep friendships I would never have had anywhere else.

Where else would you get to stand for a photo shoot with Ian McShane (remember Lovejoy?) in Covent Garden at 7am, wearing a Breast Cancer Care nightshirt? Or be interviewed live on Talk Radio by Lorraine Kelly (who, by the way, is as mad as a box of very mad frogs behind the scenes!)? How else could I ever have manifested a chat with my all-time pop hero Annie Lennox than at a benefit concert to raise money and awareness for Breast Cancer Care? (See Chapter 3 for more details.)

New Cancer, Old Lessons

Fast forward almost five years to September 1998, not long past my first wedding anniversary and heading for the magical five-year post-diagnosis milestone. Over the summer I had been thinking about how I might celebrate, or at least mark the big event. I was working in Silicon Valley, California, delivering appraisal training in the American office of my then employer. This was the only positive thing I remember about that job!

While there I took the opportunity to visit friends in my 'spiritual' home town of San Diego. As I had traveled to California in work mode, not vacation mode, I hadn't thought about packing the usual staple products, like sunscreen, for example. As a result I ended up very sunburnt on the backs of my legs. One mole reacted to the sun by becoming hard and swollen. Although I didn't worry unduly, it did remind me to make an appointment with my GP upon my return.

If there were ever proof things happen for a reason, this was it. In the same way that moving back to the UK led me to relate my medical history to a new doctor, that trip to California led me to experience the sunburn on my legs, which motivated me to get it checked out by the GP. The fact my GP responded as he did, in a very patronizing and high-handed manner, was quite possibly the single most important step in my second cancer survival! Had he taken my concern seriously and put my mind at rest, I may well not be here now, and my Post-Traumatic Success journey might have ended some years ago.

The patronizing response triggered something in me, which led me to feel indignant that I wasn't being taken seriously and was missing something to which I was entitled. Insisting on a second opinion on this occasion probably saved my life. On September 16, 1998 I received my second bombshell in five years: I was diagnosed with a malignant melanoma on my left calf.

Although it was another early diagnosis as regards the extent of the cancer's spread, this diagnosis hit me much harder at an emotional level. Still as determined as before that I was meant to use the experience to help others, I found it much harder this time to get past the 'why me?' phase. A powerful mix of guilt that I had brought this on myself through years of irresponsible sunbathing and 'woe is me' victim feeling overwhelmed me for several weeks.

The seven weeks of enforced solitary confinement (on the couch) following my surgery was one of the best and the worst times of my life, all rolled into one. It was easily the worst time up to that point in my life, as I fell into an acute state of depression about my lot. On the positive side, it was an important time for the thinking and learning opportunity it provided for me.

The learning came like a bolt from the blue, a spiritual vision almost. You see, for six weeks I just lay on the couch, my left leg elevated to allow the wound to heal and the skin graft to do its thing. I lay on the couch wondering how I had gotten myself into this position, and I *don't* mean the cancer. The cancer itself was actually the least of my worries. I had a frame of reference that I could survive cancer.

I had been working in a job for the past nine months that had been making me feel increasingly more miserable, disempowered and useless by the day. The role had not been clearly defined from the start, my manager was pulled in so many different directions by her board colleagues, I always felt I was the smallest, quietest child in a huge family, the child that was never listened to or taken seriously. During the nine months I had allowed my self-esteem and self-worth to be well and truly eroded to the core.

Can you imagine: having rolled out the company's first real appraisal process and conducted training in how to carry out a good appraisal, I eventually had my own appraisal *on the phone while driving around the M25*! My own boss provided me with my 'worst case scenario' case study, which I have used as a 'how not to…' example for the past 15 years in my training workshops!

(If you are a police or traffic officer reading this, it was 1998 and it was still legally acceptable to hold your cell phone while driving!)

I still had the overwhelming feeling and belief that I was meant to be using my traumatic experiences to help others. The experience with my cell phone appraisal was a stark reminder that I was not doing anything that made me feel useful or empowered, and I certainly wasn't following my Post-Traumatic Success path. These thoughts and feelings consumed

me during my convalescence, although it was to be
another few years before I started my personal development journey in earnest.

New Trauma, New Lessons

In 2001, during my second pregnancy, I discovered my
husband was having an affair. He denied it of course,
but I knew. I even knew who it was. I didn't have any
tangible evidence in the form of lipstick on the col-
lar, hotel receipts, hushed phone calls that end when
you enter the room, or any of the usual suspects. But
I knew. I was devastated, completely lost. This was
the man I called my soul mate, the man who stood
by my side through my worst nightmares. The man
I was having another baby with, at some risk to my
own health; the man I went out on a limb for with
my family. They had never trusted him from the start,
but were happy that he had given me a much-wanted
distraction during my cancer journeys. For this reason
alone, they were prepared to suspend their judgment
and welcome him into the family.

I felt completely helpless, once again. By comparison
with a simple cancer diagnosis, this trauma seemed
insurmountable. I felt I had no trump cards in my
hands at all. Unlike with both cancers, where I could
read up on the 'enemy' within my body, and empow-
er myself with knowledge, there seemed little help in
the text books when it came to winning your husband
back when you looked the size of a house and felt con-

stantly sick. I felt utterly alone with this trauma. This time I didn't have him on my side.

A while after the birth, when I got the tangible evidence that made it all real, I tried all the usual strategies: the crying, the shouting and screaming, the begging, the silent treatment, the 'I'm better than this', the 'I can do this on my own', the 'you've ruined my life' routines. None of them seemed to help. I ate nothing at all for three weeks and lost over 30 pounds in weight. All my baby weight and quite a lot more just melted away. At the time I saw this as a positive side-effect.

Eventually I picked myself up from this traumatic event too, and determined to look for the aspects of this situation I could take some control over. After all, the stakes were higher this time: I had two children still in diapers who were depending on me, and no soul mate to share the burden with. It was clear I could not control the external event, the affair, the decision my husband made to leave the family home and make a new life with his mistress. I therefore faced the choice I had faced twice before in the past 10 years: to sit in a corner and wait for circumstances to envelope me and take over my soul, or stand up and choose to control my experience of events.

I chose the latter. It did not feel like I had a choice at the time, I did what came naturally. In fact it was to be a good few years before I understood the full impact of my choices in those 'trauma years'. It has been much more recently that I have realized just how much my choices have made me different from many others facing similar situations.

CHAPTER 2

"It's not how far you fall,
but how high you bounce that counts."

Zig Ziglar

Why 'Post-Traumatic Success'?

If you have experienced a traumatic event – the loss of a loved one, life-threatening illness, or divorce, for example – you probably went through a number of very different emotions in the period after the event itself. Aside from physical pain, you may well have experienced anger, isolation or fear about the future as you processed what had happened to you. Indeed, many people find these emotions may be interspersed with periods where they forget or act as if the event never happened at all. Everyone's experience is different, even though there is likely to be some commonality in the course of the emotional journey.

The concept of 'post-traumatic *stress*' is not new to the newspaper headlines. While the symptoms have been described by historians and observers of war since Greek and Roman times, the phrase has been used more consistently since the 1970s to describe a set of symptoms seen in people who have witnessed something extremely traumatic, such as violent death or torture. In recent years we've heard a lot about people returning from war zones displaying horrendous after-effects of modern-day warfare: nightmares, flashbacks, changed or unpredictable behavior patterns, to name a few.

For some, the trauma they have experienced is so profound and life-altering that just finding a way through their symptoms and the consequences on a day-to-day basis will fill their waking hours for a long time, even a lifetime. My heart goes out to these people and their friends and families as they seek to make sense of the hand they have been dealt. I recognize that post-traumatic stress disorder (PTSD) is an affliction, but that is not what this book is about.

This book is dedicated to those who have processed their own experience of their traumatic event and have come to accept that the status quo has changed; what used to be 'normal' is no longer normal. There is a new definition of 'normal' for them!

Definitions

Perhaps it is helpful at this point to explore the words themselves: post – traumatic – success:

Post – [prefix]: In this context, of course, 'post-' refers to something that comes *after* something else; post-operative treatment, post-war history or a post-modernist picture, for example.

Traumatic [adjective]: Comes from the noun 'trauma'. Meaning:

1. A serious injury or shock to the body, as from violence or an accident.

2. An emotional wound or shock that creates substantial lasting damage.

3. An event or situation that causes great distress and disruption.

Success [noun]: The achievement of something desired, planned, or attempted

For some, the emotional, physical and psychological distress caused by the trauma itself will consume their energy and thoughts for the rest of their lives or at least for a long time. For others, with the help of time, therapies, treatments and plenty of support, they will come to a new and more fruitful stage in their healing, where they realize that the event itself has provided an opportunity for change.

From Stress to Success

I remember when I went through my breast cancer treatment I got to a stage quite early on, while I was still undergoing daily radiotherapy, where I wanted to use my experience to help others. In fact some might say I was desperate to do so. The physical pain from the surgery was gone, and even before I had started my personal development journey, something inside my head told me that I had gone through this experience for a reason, and the reason, I decided, was that

I had to give back to others going through the same trauma.

Of course, I wasn't *really* ready at all. Before you think I am embellishing my own experiences, or sanitizing how I remember that time – cleaning up the nostalgia, so to speak – what I was really doing was looking outside myself for distraction to avoid thinking about and processing my own trauma. Helping others is a worthy distraction, however not helpful when you have not yet worked on yourself. I was far from ready or safe to be let loose on other unsuspecting breast cancer sufferers. It's a pattern I have noticed in myself many times since then: the desire to lose myself in activity that will help others and importantly will allow me to avoid focusing on my own journey. In the management world it is often called 'displacement activity' – the activity undertaken to make procrastination feel more acceptable.

Thankfully I was being supported at the time by a fabulous breast care nurse at Cheltenham General Hospital by the name of Sue Kendall, who recognized my displacement and distraction tactics. Sue encouraged me gently (and sometimes less gently) to focus on my own healing first. She provided a listening ear, but more importantly she was also the wise voice of the impartial coach or mentor. Sue leveled with me, she told me when she thought I was wrong, and on occasion it was Sue who said the unsayable. The first two years post-diagnosis were critical in establishing that the cancer was all gone and I would not suffer a local recurrence. I could not use volunteering as a crutch or a way of meeting my own needs.

When she eventually put me in touch with the volunteer section at Breast Cancer Care two years later, I was accepted straight on to the volunteer program and underwent my training without looking back. I can't even begin to imagine how dangerous I might have been as a peer supporter in those early days, barely into the post-traumatic stage myself, and careering gung-ho into other people's lives.

The '*success*' part of this journey can only evolve when we have come through and properly processed our own post-traumatic symptoms and the consequences of the trauma on our own lives. That doesn't mean we must be 'healed'; it does mean, however, that we have taken time to understand our own trauma, and begun to draw some of the lessons *for ourselves*. I believe we need to have passed through (and recognized the passing of) our own denial and misplaced anger (see The Grieving Process below) before we can take a more balanced view of the event itself.

A loose cannon is a dangerous weapon; a loose cannon that is *in denial* or *angry* can do untold damage to anyone or anything in its sights!

Each trauma represents a form of loss or bereavement; it could be the actual loss of a loved one, or the loss of certainty, of carefree innocence or of blissful ignorance about such events. As with any loss or bereavement, there must be a period of mourning or grieving for that loss before the bereaved person is able to move on and accept the new reality (without the person or thing that has been lost).

Fear of Loss

Generally speaking, we humans are motivated more by a fear of loss or scarcity than a hope for abundance or something good. For some, the fear of loss/scarcity can be quite overwhelming, and can paralyze us in our everyday lives. Most of us make irrational decisions every day simply to avoid losing or lacking.

We might buy things we don't need (or collect coupons we won't use) because a sale is ending soon. We may allow ourselves to be seduced by two-for-one offers and time-limited deals, or we grab an item of clothing because there's only one left and someone else might take it – even if we aren't really sure we want it.

And that's not all. People turn down all sorts of opportunities every day that could be beneficial to avoid the risk of losing something else they convince themselves is good enough. We use our time in ways that feel unfulfilling because we fear losing time on a decision that might be wrong. For example, we might spend hours and hours working on an admin task, learning a software product to create something which we might otherwise outsource for a fraction of the cost of our time.

There's a big fear of loss that I come across in my work on a daily basis: many, many people think twice (or three times) about investing in themselves, even though they desperately want to expand their mind, their opportunities and their options, purely because it can feel painful or just wrong to part with money on something for themselves. They measure the loss or lack of the money in the bank over the investment in their own mind, or education, which could ultimately bring benefit and abundance to their whole family.

The Grieving Process

Elisabeth Kübler Ross (1926-2004), a psychiatrist who worked extensively with people suffering life-threatening illness, recognized that they all go through a process when they are first given the news, until they are finally able to accept what is happening and move on. While the whole process is an opportunity to learn from the traumatic event, it is only at the stage of acceptance that we can really start considering how we might turn the experience into something more meaningful and positive – *success,* in other words.

It was as a result of her work with the dying that Elisabeth Kübler Ross formulated the Grief Curve, which has been quoted, misquoted and embellished many times since its origins in the 1960s. The original Grief Curve has frequently been adapted as a management model and renamed the Change Curve or the Transition Curve, and is used to describe the process an employee goes through when faced with unwanted change, such as redundancy or changes to the working environment. In effect, an employee facing redundancy or changes to his/her contract goes through a grieving process, mourning the loss of financial certainty or perhaps the loss of trust in the employer.

Kübler Ross identified five distinct phases in the grieving process:

1. **Denial** – 'I feel fine.'; 'This can't be happening, not to me.'

2. **Anger** – 'Why me? It's not fair!'; 'How can this happen to me?'; 'Who is to blame?'

3. **Bargaining** – 'I'll do anything for a few more years.'; 'I will give my life savings if...'

4. **Depression** – 'I'm so sad, why bother with anything?'; 'I'm going to die soon so what's the point?'; 'I miss my loved one, why go on?'

5. **Acceptance** – 'It's going to be okay.'; 'I can't fight it, I may as well prepare for it.'

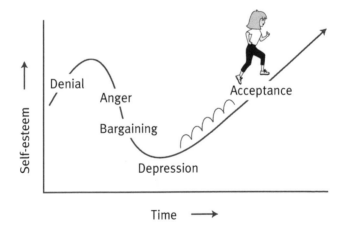

Over the years I have worked with many clients who have created their ideas for their own Post-Traumatic

Success at Phase 3 in their journey: Bargaining. It is not unknown for people to try to broker a deal with God or their faith, or perhaps with the Universe, along the lines of 'I swear I'll set up a hospice for the starving orphans of Ethiopia if I survive this', and to achieve this feat against the odds.

Well, we're now a few pages into this book, so it must be time for an exercise!

Exercise: Understanding Your Grief Curve

As you reflect on Elisabeth Kübler Ross's Grief Curve, write down some of the emotions, feelings and thoughts you experienced at each of the stages of the grieving process. These questions might help you:

- *Think back to each stage in the aftermath of your traumatic event; what words describe how you felt in each phase?*

- *What do you remember thinking in each phase?*

- *What did you say? Can you remember verbatim anything you might have said to friends or posted in your Facebook status at the time?*

- *How did each phase of the process manifest itself for you?*

- *How long did each phase last?*

- *How did you know you were moving on to the next phase?*

- *Did you find yourself going back and forth between two different phases? How long did that last?*

- *What did you do to support and look after yourself at each phase?*

- ...

The Only Reality is Now

A model, however accurate, is still only a model. At best it is a useful two-dimensional representation to help you understand or explain what may be happening for you as you experience your post-traumatic emotions and thoughts.

What is real, however, is the here and now, how you are feeling, what you are seeing, hearing, experiencing in the present. I meet many people who say: "I understand the Grief Curve, I don't understand why I'm not experiencing... " or "It's been six months since the accident, I should be feeling... by now."

'Should' or 'ought' language is not helpful; everyone's experience of the same situation is different. Take a car accident, for example, or a fight in a bar on a Saturday night; each witness will experience the accident or the fight differently depending on where they were standing, at what angle they were viewing the action, and of course their relationship with the parties involved. In fact, if you *are* one of the parties involved, you'll have a different experience of the event altogether. In effect there is no such thing as 'reality', reality is each person's perception. It's why we pay lawyers such large fees to represent our perceptions of reality in court.

'Should' language suggests the language of a critical parent: 'you *should* put a coat on, it's cold outside' or 'you *should* start saving for a pension so you have enough money to retire one day'. If we use 'should' language with ourselves, we may well find this engenders emotional responses to what we *should* be experiencing, piled on top of what we are actually experiencing! When we convince ourselves that we should do or feel a certain thing, this may bring feelings of guilt to the surface – guilt that we are not feeling or behaving as we *should*.

The vital message here is **there is no wrong way to feel**! Some people bounce back from a traumatic event faster than others, some need longer to work through their own post-traumatic process. Some cry and scream and throw things, others become quiet and withdrawn. There's no 'should' about any of it, that's just the way it is.

Survivor Guilt

There is a phenomenon which has been well documented in management literature as well as health journals and books: this is the feeling of guilt at having survived or come off lightly compared with others. Survivor guilt as a human mental health condition was first identified during the 1960s; over time several therapists have linked the symptoms to Holocaust survivors. More recently the condition tends to be attributed to survivors of traumatic situations such as war, natural disasters, and even among the friends and family of suicide victims.

At a psychological level, a person suffering from survivor guilt might feel shame, sad, powerless, helpless or worthless; they question why they deserved to survive when others did not. In the corporate world, managers recognize the phenomenon in teams that remain where there have been redundancies. Even where there is no obvious danger to human life, the symptoms can be equally bewildering, debilitating and ultimately life-altering for the individuals affected.

For some people undoubtedly, it is this survivor guilt that galvanizes them to set out on their Post-Traumatic Success journey.

The Most Destructive Four-Letter Word Ever

I had a very profound experience of this during my basic training to become a volunteer with Breast Cancer Care, all over a seemingly trivial four-letter word. No, it's *not* the one you're thinking! I remember being in the room with 13 other volunteer rookies as we sat expectantly one Saturday morning in November 1995. At this stage we had not yet gotten to know each other or formed a bond. We had arrived on the Friday night, and had been allocated our twin bedrooms which we were asked to share with another trainee volunteer. I had met my bedroom buddy, but that was it, the other 12 women in the room were complete strangers.

It was a very odd situation; having attended many, many seminars, workshops and conferences since then, the idea of buddying up and sharing a room with a complete stranger to minimize costs no longer holds quite the fear it did then. You know that if nothing else, you have a shared interest in the topic of the workshop. Added to that, it is likely these days that you have also corresponded with your prospective bedroom buddy by email, Facebook, text or shared forum beforehand.

Back on that cold frosty Saturday morning in November 1995, I didn't know any of these women from Adam (or Eve, for that matter!). All I knew was they had all survived breast cancer at least two years earlier. That in itself is quite an icebreaker, it turns out!

The workshop started in the traditional way – health and safety briefing, directions to the bathrooms and general housekeeping for the day, followed by introductions around the room. Each woman was invited to introduce herself by sharing as much of her own story as she was comfortable sharing. As the stories were released into the room, three things struck me about the stories and their owners:

1. All the women in the room were significantly older than me (I was 34).

2. Every woman's experience of her own breast cancer journey was different – her emotions, her symptoms, her fears and beliefs, and above all the decisions she had made.

3. Every woman in the room seemed to have had much more aggressive treatment than I had (most had had mastectomies), much more debilitating side-effects, more pain, more drugs, a worse prognosis – and in my head, therefore, were *much* more justified in being there than I was!

The introductions finally got around to me. I really wished I'd been asked to go first, then the other women in the room might have forgotten just how easy a time I had had with my diagnosis and treatment.

"Hello, my name is Diana Whitehead, I'm 34 years old and I… only had a lumpectomy followed by radiothera...' I ventured, somewhat apologetically.

"Excuse me!" boomed the hitherto sweet voice of the trainer at the front. "What is the meaning of *'ONLY'*? This is not a competition, you know! How many other 34-year-olds do you know who have been treated for breast cancer?"

Well, the room fell silent. I was suddenly aware of 14 pairs of eyes trained on me like well-honed snipers from all around the horseshoe, as well as from the petite, unassuming trainer at the front. Any hopes I may have harbored to keep a low profile and tuck myself into a corner for the weekend were now well and truly out the window!

I learned a very profound lesson on that cold frosty November morning in that budget hotel room in London: I learned how destructive that four-letter word 'only' can be to one's confidence, self-esteem, and one's whole identity of oneself. In trying to fit in by comparing my experience of this horrible disease unfavorably with that of others in the room, I was questioning, even dismissing as less valid, my experience of my own experience. I actually felt *guilty* for having gone through a less traumatic treatment regime for a disease that kills millions of people every year!

Since that November day I have caught myself doing the *'only'* thing to myself many times over. The difference now is that I do catch myself doing it, and remind myself of that esteem-building lesson all those years ago. I'm sure the trainer did not realize the profound impact she had, not only on my life that day but also on the lives of the many clients I have coached and supported over the years doing the *'only'* thing to themselves.

Locus of Control

While comparison is clearly not a helpful activity when talking about our experience of traumatic events, as demonstrated by the 'only' example above, I am nevertheless interested in how we as human beings differ in our approach to, and our resilience in, the face of trauma. Let's face it, we all know of people who seem to lurch through life from one crisis to the next, with some seeming to take these in their stride better than others.

Why is it, for example, that some people seem to be dealt a tough hand in this life, with one drama following another, and seem to have ways of coping better than others who have no problems by comparison? We probably all know someone within our circle of friends, or in the neighborhood, who has had to deal with health complications, job loss, relationship crises, only to go on to have a child with some emotional or physical challenges. Somehow that person takes what is dealt to them with grace, or at least with a level of acceptance we might find difficult to understand. Conversely we probably all know the person who always has something to gripe about, the person who can create a drama out of a mild inconvenience and who also needs to tell everyone about it.

Research has shown that *locus of control* plays an important role in determining the control one perceives to have over oneself and events. *Locus of Control* was first conceptualized by John Rotter (1966). He discovered that those who believe they can make choices to determine or take control over their own circumstances have what he called an *internal locus of control*, while those who believe their circumstances are controlled by external forces or other people have an *external locus of control*. Many who have an *external locus of control* are more prone to stress, and may suffer from depression during their lives, particularly as a result of a traumatic event. One study showed that participants who had more of an *internal locus of control* had a better chance of making a commitment to change, whereas the participants who had more of an *external locus of control* were found to have more difficulty committing to change in their lives.

Further studies have shown that those who experience trauma have positive attributes such as an increased sense of self-confidence, an increased connection to others, and an enhanced sense of the meaning of life. Those who can make sense of their loss and feel in control of it are generally more likely to adjust more easily to their changed post-traumatic circumstances.

Suzanne Kobasa took the concept of *locus of control* a stage further in the late 1970s and researched what she called *psychological hardiness*, particularly in managers in the corporate world and their ability to cope with stress in the workplace. She discovered that individuals who scored highly in *psychological hardiness* (which we might equate to an *internal locus of control*) seemed to react to stressful events by interacting with them and trying to turn them into an advantage and opportunity for growth, and in the process achieve some greater understanding.

What would be interesting would be to measure the *locus of control* in those of us who are determined to follow our Post-Traumatic Success journey, come hell or high water. I'd like to offer you that opportunity right now.

Exercise: Your Locus of Control

For each question select the statement that you agree with the most:

1. a. Children get into trouble because their parents punish them too much.

    b. The trouble with most children nowadays is that their parents are too easy with them.

2. a. Many of the unhappy things in people's lives are partly due to bad luck.

    b. People's misfortunes result from the mistakes they make.

3. a. One of the major reasons why we have wars is because people don't take enough interest in politics.

    b. There will always be wars, no matter how hard people try to prevent them.

4. a. In the long run people get the respect they deserve in this world.

    b. Unfortunately, an individual's worth often passes unrecognized no matter how hard he tries.

5. a. The idea that teachers are unfair to students is nonsense.

    b. Most students don't realize the extent to which their grades are influenced by accidental happenings.

6. a. Without the right breaks one cannot be an effective leader.

   b. Capable people who fail to become leaders have not taken advantage of their opportunities.

7. a. No matter how hard you try, some people just don't like you.

   b. People who can't get others to like them don't understand how to get along with others.

8. a. Heredity plays the major role in determining one's personality.

   b. It is one's experiences in life which determine what people are like.

9. a. I have often found that what is going to happen will happen.

   b. Trusting to fate has never turned out as well for me as making a decision to take a definite course of action.

10. a. In the case of the well-prepared student there is rarely if ever such a thing as an unfair test.

    b. Many times exam questions tend to be so unrelated to course work that studying is really useless.

11. a. Becoming a success is a matter of hard work; luck has little or nothing to do with it.

b. Getting a good job depends mainly on being in the right place at the right time.

12. a. The average citizen can have an influence in government decisions.

b. This world is run by the few people in power, and there is not much the little guy can do about it.

13. a. When I make plans, I am almost certain that I can make them work.

b. It is not always wise to plan too far ahead because many things turn out to be a matter of good or bad fortune anyhow.

14. a. There are certain people who are just no good.

b. There is some good in everybody.

15. a. In my case getting what I want has little or nothing to do with luck.

b. Many times we might just as well decide what to do by flipping a coin.

16. a. Who gets to be the boss often depends on who was lucky enough to be in the right place first.

b. Getting people to do the right thing depends upon ability; luck has little or nothing to do with it.

17. a. As far as world affairs are concerned, most of us are the victims of forces we can neither understand nor control.

    b. By taking an active part in political and social affairs, the people can control world events.

18. a. Most people don't realize the extent to which their lives are controlled by accidental happenings.

    b. There really is no such thing as luck.

19. a. One should always be willing to admit mistakes.

    b. It is usually best to cover up one's mistakes.

20. a. It is hard to know whether or not a person really likes you.

    b. How many friends you have depends upon how nice a person you are.

21. a. In the long run the bad things that happen to us are balanced by the good ones.

    b. Most misfortunes are the result of lack of ability, ignorance, laziness, or all three.

22. a. With enough effort we can wipe out political corruption.

    b. It is difficult for people to have much control over the things politicians do in office.

23. a. Sometimes I can't understand how teachers arrive at the grades they give.

b. There is a direct connection between how hard I study and the grades I get.

24. a. A good leader expects people to decide for them selves what they should do.

b. A good leader makes it clear to everybody what their jobs are.

25. a. Many times I feel I have little influence over the things that happen to me.

b. It is impossible for me to believe that chance or luck plays an important role in my life.

26. a. People are lonely because they don't try to be friendly.

b. There's not much use in trying too hard to please people; if they like you, they like you.

27. a. There is too much emphasis on athletics in high school.

b. Team sports are an excellent way to build character.

28. a. What happens to me is my own doing.

b. Sometimes I feel that I don't have enough control over the direction my life is taking.

29. a. Most of the time I can't understand why politicians behave the way they do.

b. In the long run the people are responsible for bad government on a national as well as on a local level.

Score one point for each of the following:

1.	11. b	21. a
2. a	12. b	22. b
3. b	13. b	23. a
4. b	14.	24.
5. b	15. b	25.a
6. a	16. a	26. b
7. a	17. a	27.
8.	18. a	28. b
9. a	19.	29. a
10. b	20. a	

A high score = External Locus of Control

A low score = Internal Locus of Control

Note: Some statements are inserted as the control study and are therefore not scored.

So Am I the Victim or the Victor?

I heard a hypothesis many years ago, after both my touches with cancer and before I had ever heard of the *locus of control*, which gave me a new perspective on my own experiences and those of others. In fact this hypothesis has allowed me to make huge changes, not only in how I viewed my own traumatic events, but also in the types of experiences I have actively sought out since then.

The hypothesis was this: that every traumatic event in life is 'sent' as an opportunity to learn a lesson we need to learn in life. We are only sent those lessons we need and are able to learn, and it is up to us to work out what that lesson is, and how best to learn it. We don't have to do this alone; in fact more often than not, learning can be not only more enjoyable but more memorable, profound and more life-enhancing if we learn alongside someone who can support us – a mentor, coach or therapist, for example.

'So what about those people who have several bad things happen to them? Are you saying they have more to learn?' I hear you cry. Here's the thing: when we receive the lesson (or 'learning opportunity' if that's not too patronizing an expression), we have choices. One choice is to reject the learning outright and carry on as if nothing had changed; think about those people who succumb to a heart attack or a stroke, and carry on smoking, drinking or eating food that is compromising their recovery. Another choice is to sink so deep into a victim mentality that we might miss the learning altogether.

I have worked with many women who have thought of themselves as a victim to their breast cancer; they are the unfortunate one, the one who has lived the virtuous life, only to fall victim to this cruel killer. These may be women of whom others ask, 'Why do bad things happen to good people?' Some may spiral into these unhelpful victim thoughts and emotions for years and years, fueled and encouraged in this vortex of disempowerment and negativity by those well-meaning friends and colleagues around them who say things like 'What did she ever do to deserve this?'

Meeting people who have been sucked into such a maelstrom of 'poor me' throughout the last 20 years is one of the main reasons this book has come into being.

I realize that's rather a grandiose statement to be making, and yet it needs to be said. I have worked with, lived near, and spoken on the bus with people disillusioned with their jobs, upset at being made redundant, even people who have suffered serious illness, car accidents, heart attacks, or violence at the hands of others, who have spent years perfecting the pose, the speech, the alter ego of The Victim, almost like rehearsing for the lead role in a Broadway or West End play!

Despite all my work as a counselor, coach and friend, I still find it difficult to empathize truly with the 'victim' role. As I think back to the difficult events that have shaped my life, they seem to have slotted in, found their place in the rich tapestry, as things that needed to be navigated, much like roundabouts or speed bumps in the road. Now I'm not saying this to sound holier than thou, in fact I waited for those victim thoughts and emotions to come in the days, weeks and months following the traumatic events in my life. But they never did. In case you were wondering, I'm not Superwoman or Pollyanna! I certainly experienced (and still do) deeply negative emotions such as anger, paralyzing fear, sadness, even vengefulness at times. I'm human, after all!

The problem I have with being a victim is that it feels as though I would need to look outside for a solution, a way out. It feels like a place of unresourcefulness, a place of total surrender (or sell-out) to external circumstances or people. One pattern I recognize very clearly in myself is that, when pushed into a corner by a negative or difficult event, after a short period of licking my wounds, I regroup. I get resourceful. I think about who or what could help me now: where could I go to get new information, what have I done before in a similar situation?

My mantra in such situations is 'It ain't over till the fat lady sings'!

And aside from the occasional visit to the opera, I don't tend to spend too much time around singing fat ladies!

I learned a question in the very early days of my neuro-linguistic programing (NLP) training which is with me all the time, and serves me in times of self-pity: 'What if you could…?'

- What if you could find the money to pay this bill?

- What if you could persuade the client to buy your training program?

- What if you could find childcare and go to the party on Saturday?

- What if you could find an alternative therapy that might help with the pain?

- What if you could make it on your own following the relationship breakdown?

- What if you could start your own business after redundancy?

- What if you could afford your dream vacation, house, car, etc.?

- What if you could find a way to hire a cleaner?

The last one probably reveals more about me than it should!

Delayed Learning?

If every experience in life is a learning opportunity, how do I know what I'm supposed to learn? What if I don't get the lesson, and therefore miss the learning? What if I already 'know' that lesson, do I have to attend the class again?

The idea that traumatic events are learning opportunities throws up many more questions than it answers. The thing about learning is that it is not always linear or instantaneous; sometimes you go through the lesson and reflect later, when it's all over. Some people only put two and two together months or even years later with the help of an experienced counselor or guide.

If there is some truth in it, perhaps it explains why some people seem to go through traumatic event after traumatic event in their lives. Perhaps they have more to learn, or at least have a greater capacity to learn from these events, or perhaps they missed an opportunity to learn the lesson the first time around, and so have another opportunity in the 'revision class'. (I hate to use the 1970s term 'remedial class' although it has felt like that for me on occasion!)

In reality there is probably some truth in both of these. I had the opportunity to reflect after my breast cancer diagnosis, although I was so keen to get back to some sense of 'normal' or certainty, I skated over the opportunities provided to me by the experience, and instead took a few short cuts along the way. I reflected, for example, on what might have caused the cancer; I ate a pretty healthy diet (I was a vegetarian following a bout of salmonella three years earlier thanks to a very expensive veal steak in a high-class restaurant in Konstanz, Southern Germany, which put me right off meat) and up to my diagnosis had played squash two or three times a week – enthusiastically and regularly, if not competitively or very well!

When my breast cancer was diagnosed I had been back in the UK for three months, having lived and worked in Germany for 11 years before that. I had just completed the first semester of a very intensive (and expensive) MBA (Master's degree in Business Administration) at Warwick Business School, and once I knew the surgery had been successful (successful meaning I had woken up after the anesthetic), I was keen to get back to the course I had invested so heavily in, without further delay.

So, after some initial reflection on a thesis I had read about cancer being caused by emotional stress, I made an unconscious decision to postpone my learning until after the MBA. After all, I had enough learning on my plate with the business, economics and marketing themes and the exams I had to study for. I put off dealing with the emotional roller coaster and focused on getting back into attending lectures and writing assignments just one week after leaving hospital.

While I was 'successful' by others' standards during that time, for me there was always something missing. Awarded an MBA with Distinction at the end of 1994 put me into the top 10% of MBA students graduating from Warwick Business School (WBS was No. 1 in the league of business schools in the UK at that time), and I didn't feel successful! While I enjoyed the graduation ceremony and seeing all my fellow students again, I couldn't help that niggling thought in the back of my mind that this wasn't real success, that there must be something more than this.

That in itself made me feel all the more different and freakish. In reality, my own Post-Traumatic Success journey didn't begin for another five years, when I was diagnosed with a malignant melanoma. Another learning opportunity! And it wasn't until a few years after this event that I shared with a counselor during my divorce that I had never felt deserving of the Distinction; after all, they must have given it to me out of pity! I still had a lot to learn on my post-traumatic journey!

CHAPTER 3

"A bridge of silver wings stretches from the dead ashes
of an unforgiving nightmare to the jeweled vision
of a life started anew."
Aberjhani, *The River of Winged Dreams*

Design Your Post-Traumatic Success CREATION

It's always intrigued me that some people seem to have come out of the womb with a destiny, knowing exactly what they were put on this earth to do. They travel through childhood on the trajectory that will take them to their destined career – be that train driver, actor or nuclear physicist. Perhaps you were one of those people? When family or your parents' friends came to visit and asked the time-tested 'what do you want to be when you grow up?', were you one of those children who knew from an early age what they wanted to do? And have you actually followed it through?

I suspect (and hope) I belong to the majority of people who had no idea what they wanted to be when they grew up, and for whom a career path sort of materializes during high school, born out of an interest in certain subjects and the obligatory chats with the careers advisors at school.

I remember the careers advisor at my school advising me to consider a career in the forces – the Royal Navy, for example – where I'd be able to combine my language skills and interest in sailing. As I think back over the 35 or so years since that conversation took place, I can smile at the inappropriateness of the advice. Someone less likely to follow rules and instructions would be hard to find! In fact I seek out rules just so I can bend them, in all areas of life. I enjoy the thrill of successfully challenging a parking ticket, so much so I do it for friends too!

(If you are a traffic officer or police officer reading this, of course I keep within the law as a road user at all times, and I merely challenge where I strongly believe the officer has made a genuine mistake!)

Feeling Different

I didn't have a clue what I wanted to be when I grew up, the whole way through school. The only thing I knew then, and still feel now as I mentioned in Chapter 1, is that I always felt different from others. I never really felt like I fitted in, and the careers advice at school confirmed that for me. It transpired I couldn't join the forces for two reasons that made me different: firstly I wore contact lenses (I was the first in my school to do so) and secondly I hold a US passport alongside my British one, so this would have precluded me. I must say, I was relieved at the time, as I couldn't really see myself in a uniform, following instructions or even giving instructions to others.

The alternative careers advice I was given was hotel and catering management. Indeed French, German and Home Economics 'A' levels might well lead a careers advisor to this conclusion; however, again I remained unconvinced. To be honest I probably didn't really know what it entailed, never having stayed in a hotel at that point.

I knew of myself that I enjoyed having people around me, lots of people. I never really had a best friend throughout my school days, partly a result of moving around from school to school as the family moved for my dad's work. I was always one of the crowd, the joker or entertainer of the crowd. I see the same traits in my son Laurence now, surrounded by friends, no special best friend, but always the one playing the fool. The jury's out as to whether this is a good gene to have passed on, since it tends to come with the pitfall of being caught out by teachers on a regular basis!

The feeling of being different from everyone else manifested itself in all sorts of areas; we were the only family I knew with a dog, for example. In fact we had two for many years. It was always difficult when friends came to the house as many of my friends were afraid of dogs, so we would first have to shut the dogs away before people could come in. Also most of my friends' mums didn't work, or worked part-time, so they were home when my friends got home from school. I was the first latchkey kid of all my friends.

Now I don't say any of this to complain or whinge about my terrible childhood, in fact quite the opposite;

I was the first of my friends to go abroad on vacation. Thinking about it now, I'm sure there's a link between having a working mum and enjoying foreign vacations! The fact that I already felt different stood me in good stead when I was the first of my friends to be diagnosed with breast cancer, the first to be divorced, even the first person I knew to have children after breast cancer. I already felt different as a child, so that was not a lesson I needed to learn in adulthood.

Making Different Choices

By feeling different from others, it is not such a big leap to find yourself acting differently, taking different decisions and seeking out others who feel different. When I declared to the breast care nurse at the hospital that I wanted to help other women who were going through the same as me, it seemed the most natural thing in the world, in *my* world at least. Although I did not know then what I know now, I had a feeling I was meant to use the experience positively. I felt the experience would gain some meaning or purpose for me if I could use it to help others.

While Sue, the breast care nurse, calmly told me it was too soon, my family were rather more vocal in their reactions. "Why would you want to surround yourself with sick people?" they asked. "Concentrate on getting well yourself." The point was, I saw that as an important part of getting well myself! I was a little exasperated, though not surprised given my 'different-ness', that they could not see this.

So what does this mean for you? If you have come through a traumatic experience, do you feel different from others? Did you feel different before this happened, or has the feeling only started since the event? It doesn't really matter which came first; the feeling different or the traumatic life event; the important point is what do you want to *do* about it? Will it be a small change or a HUGE one? Do you want to make some shifts in your diet or exercise regime to increase your fitness level or are you going out to change the world and rid the planet of poverty?

However insignificant or HUGE you perceive the change you want to make, the important question now is WHEN are you going to start?

It's very easy to put things off to tomorrow, until there is better weather, until I'm feeling better, until I've attended one more training course, until I'm a bit more financially secure… I should know, I've said them all! I wrote the manual for most of them! The point is, when will tomorrow come? When will the horizon get closer? Putting things off till tomorrow is like looking out to the horizon, to a time where things will be better, the stars will be aligned and that will be the right time to start a business, take up running, write a book (!) or whatever it is.

So when will the horizon get closer? The answer is the horizon NEVER gets any closer, it's always in the same place, it's as far away as the eye can see. It's where our pre-Galileo ancestors assumed the edge of the flat earth to be.

It'll be time for another exercise shortly, but first here's a model you may have come across if you work in the corporate world and have attended any training workshops:

Johari Window

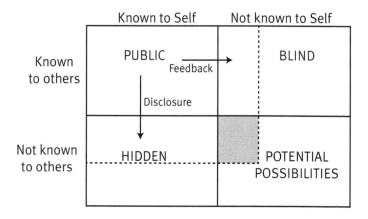

In this model your Public window (top left) is just that – the things about you that are in the public domain. This is particularly true if you consider things you are vocal about; these might be things such as:

- Your attitude toward smokers, non-smokers, fat people, thin people, managers, non-managers, people who watch *Big Brother* or *Newsnight*

- How confident you feel about public speaking

- How well you speak a foreign language

- Your preference for tea or coffee

The bottom right box is your Potential or Possibilities box; this is where anything is possible as the things in this box are unknown to either you or anyone else. What could be hiding in that box that could be helpful on your journey to your own Post-Traumatic Success, I wonder? Could you be the next great classical pianist or Paralympic bungee jumper? (I'm not sure that is an Olympic sport yet, but it might become one!) Could you discover the cure for snoring or does your success lie more in the area of an ambition you want to achieve for yourself: climbing to Base Camp on Everest, for example, or appearing in the *Guinness Book of Records* for the largest collection of pet guinea pigs?

The world is your oyster in the Potential box. I sometimes call this Pandora's Box – will you have the curiosity and the courage to open it? And when you do, what will you find inside? Will you find the disease, sickness, hate and envy, the dark secrets you would not have chosen to find? Or might you just open it and find the little creature called Hope, the last to fly out in the original mythological story?

Stop 'Shoulding' All Over Yourself!

What if you don't really know what it is you were meant to learn from this traumatic event, or you're not sure what your Post-Traumatic Success 'should' be? I have clients who believe they 'should' use their experience to help others going through the same, or they 'should' do something far more altruistic with their lives. Some feel the fact they have survived the event itself means they 'should' now spend the rest of their life in a state of penance, doing good works. Some people I work with believe that surviving the event means they 'should' go out and seek adrenaline-laden experiences such as skydiving over the Grand Canyon, as if to prove they are grateful!

The thing about 'shoulding' is that it sounds rather like a critical parent inside your head, telling you what they would like you to do based on their own map of the world; you *should* put a coat on, it's cold outside, you *should* go to bed early, you *should* eat vegetables to make you big and strong… If you are feeling you should be doing something altruistic or momentous in gratitude for your post-traumatic survival, you may well find your heart is not really in it, and as a result it does not fulfill you in the way you (or others) expected it to.

Post-Traumatic Success is not about 'should', it's about what you *want* success to be. Anything else, by definition, will not be successful. What will fill you up and give meaning to the traumatic event from your perspective, not your parents', not your friends' and certainly not some 'should' perspective you have created out of survivor guilt? What will give you pleasure, enjoyment, a feeling of achievement for yourself?

Exercise: What's Your Goal?

If you are familiar with the GROW model as used by many coaches the world over, this exercise is designed to help you come up with and clearly define the G, the Goal that will lead to your Post-Traumatic Success. The following is a list of questions to help you establish what it is you want to do to give meaning to the traumatic event you have come through.

Some questions are bound to resonate with you more than others; that's fine, there is no compulsion to answer every question. This is not a 'should' exercise, after all! By merely reading the questions you will commit some or all to your subconscious mind, which will continue to turn them over, work with them, come up with possible answers and perhaps even give you a Eureka moment in the coming hours and days.

As you read through the questions, you might want to take a few notes, write down single words or phrases, maybe a picture or diagram, even start a mind map if you're familiar with those. Notice the questions or words that jump out at you, notice how they make you feel, what thoughts and pictures come into your head as you read them. Make a note of anything you notice as you do this exercise.

1. What do you want MORE of in your life? (make a list)
2. What do you want LESS of in your life? (make a list)
3. What areas of your life could be improved, upgraded or tweaked?
4. What three things are in your life currently that are not serving you?
5. What do you LOVE?

6. What do you HATE?

7. Who do you enjoy spending time with? (individuals or groups)

8. What individuals or groups would you like to spend more time with?

9. Where do you enjoy spending time? (name places, situations, activities etc.)

10. What makes you feel good?

11. Where do you get your energy from? (list the activities, people, situations that energize you)

12. What would the top five things on your 'bucket list' be?

13. If you were going to live the life you *really* desire, what's the first thing you would change?

14. What do you really *really* want?

15. For your life to be perfect, what would have to change?

16. What's one change you could make in your lifestyle that would give you more peace?

17. Complete this sentence in as many different ways as you can: 'If only...'

18. What would you do or try out if you knew you couldn't fail?

19. What could be the biggest impact from achieving this?

20. If your friends, family or complete strangers were to be interviewed about your Post-Traumatic Success, what would you like them to say?

If You Knew You Couldn't Fail... Dream BIG

You may notice the questions got bigger and bigger as the list went on. The list started with just asking you to note things you like/dislike about your life right now, and graduated to thinking much bigger toward the end. That is because many of us aspire to things that are within our comfort zone now, things that are safe and that could be achieved without too much risk.

I heard a comment recently that made me smile: 'If it's not scary, it's not big enough'! I wholeheartedly agree – after all, you've been through a traumatic event and come out the other side stronger and more resilient than before (even if it doesn't always feel like it). I bet there were moments during that time that were scary, and you're still here to tell the tale.

Walt Disney said: "If you can dream it, you can do it." So how big is your dream? Is it writing a book? Starting a new business? Running two miles, or visiting a different continent? Will it involve making more money, or getting fitter than you have ever been? Do you want to help others who are going through similar trauma to yours, or work with the starving people of Africa?

If you're going to dream, you might as well dream BIG. If you're going to go outside what is comfortable and grow your comfort zone, you might as well step right out, both feet, and really go for it on your dream. After all, as a friend said to me: "If you're scared of spiders, does it really matter how big the spider is?" She has a point; for someone who is really REALLY scared of spiders, a spider is a spider! They're really scared of ALL spiders, regardless of size!

If it's Not Scary, it's Not Big Enough!

I'm assuming by this point you've got some idea of WHAT your Post-Traumatic Success is about, perhaps what it will look like when you've achieved it, WHO it will help or serve, if appropriate, and WHY you're even contemplating it.

Good. Now I'd like you to go on a little journey with me and turn this idea into a big ol' hairy, scary spider; that's right, I'd like you to turn this into something BIG! Remember the saying 'If it's not scary, it's not big enough'? I'd like you to make your Post-Traumatic Success REALLY big and REALLY scary. Now, you might be thinking *but I've done the scary stuff, coming through the traumatic event, why would I want to scare myself voluntarily now it's over?*

Reason is, if you have a dream to use your traumatic event to change something in your life, I want to make sure that change is as great as it can be for you. I really want to help you turn your misfortune into the greatest fortune it can be (this could be financial fortune, or an internal feeling of 'I'm fortunate', it doesn't matter which). I've realized that Post-Traumatic Success for me is about helping as many people as I possibly can to achieve theirs, in a way that is far bigger than they could ever have imagined for themselves. I have confidence in you, and your ability to do this, even if you don't yet!

That sounds a bit crazy – why would I have this confidence in you when we don't even know each other very well yet? I have it because there have been people in my life – counselors, coaches, mentors, even passing acquaintances – who have had confidence in me along the way, even before I had confidence in myself. I was able to borrow that confidence (however tentatively and disbelievingly) until I had enough of my own. So, you see, I know this works. I know I can have that confidence in you because, after all, you're still here. You've survived your own traumatic event, and you've read this far, so I know you're resilient *and* still curious at the very least!

Let's say your Post-Traumatic Success dream is to write a book about your experience, or start a charity in aid of your cause. Now, you may be thinking *I'll write a book and self-publish and give a few copies away to friends and family. That way I'll be leaving a legacy for my children or for other sufferers and it'll feel good seeing my name in print.* Did you know that Elvis Presley's career started with a plastic 'disc' entitled *My Happiness* and *That's When Your Heartaches Begin* that he created as a gift for his mother's birthday? He even had to pay $3.98 for the privilege! Look where that small safe dream led!

Maybe you're thinking *I'll start a charity and raise some money for others in the same situation.* Or *I'll pick a charity and find ways to raise money or awareness for that cause.* A worthy dream, of course. That was my small comfortable dream back in 1995: to raise some money for

Breast Cancer Care and help others as they wake up to the frightening news they have breast cancer.

I Dreamed a Dream

It was at Breast Cancer Care in 1998 that I met a very impressive and dynamic lady who became a good friend for the few months our paths ran in parallel on this earth. At 38 Beth Wagstaff was a year older than me, and was undergoing aggressive treatment for breast cancer, which she already knew would kill her within a few months. I remember the first time I met her as vividly as if it were yesterday. She was bald and bloated from the chemotherapy drugs, and yet when she walked into that meeting room at Breast Cancer Care's office in Putney, it was as if a whirlwind had struck. Her energy, her enthusiasm and her no-messing effervescence were like nothing I had experienced before, and certainly not the traits you might expect to see in a dying woman.

Beth had a dream. Together with Justine Picardie, sister of the *Observer* journalist Ruth Picardie who succumbed to her own breast cancer in 1997, Beth vowed to use what time she had left to found a charity for younger women with breast cancer. Her dream, as she explained to us that day, was to raise £10,000 before she died, to be used to provide information and services for younger women with breast cancer. It was her promise to Ruth, and would be her legacy. She had already chosen the name The Lavender Trust before coming across Breast Cancer Care's Younger Women Network.

The Lavender Trust was launched on May 1, 1998, on what would have been Ruth's 34th birthday. The next day Beth and Justine stood proudly on stage at the Institute of Contemporary Arts (ICA) in London as they introduced a small intimate benefit concert for 300 close friends and acquaintances, each of whom had paid over £100 for a ticket.

Over 20 years later I can still say, hand on heart, this was one of the most memorable evenings of my life. It was the evening the Eurythmics re-formed for a one-night-only live event, and I got to meet my all-time pop hero and girl-crush, Annie Lennox. Watching her from about 10 yards away, with tears in her eyes as she sang *There Must be an Angel, Here Comes the Rain Again, When Tomorrow Comes* and *The Miracle of Love* was quite amazing. Chatting with her over a glass of champagne at the post-concert reception was other-worldly!

Also amazing and almost other-worldly was what happened at the end of the concert, when the 300 guests started to leave. Beth asked me to stand at the door with Jon, her husband, and thank people for coming. As the first couple of people made their way to the doors, I noticed people were reaching for their wallets. Despite the high ticket price, the guests wanted to do more for the cause. The first couple to reach the door asked me where the collection box was, as the husband pulled a wad of £50 notes from his wallet.

I believe that may have been the first £50 note I had ever seen.

I looked across the doorway to Jon, to see he was facing exactly the same dilemma. He shrugged his shoulders, which I took as a sign to go and find something – anything – in which to collect money. I ran as fast as I could to the box office and found an empty photocopy paper box with a lid.

Beth's dream to raise £10,000 before she died came true that night; we took over £10,000 in donations on the door from people who had already spent over £100 to be there. Over the next seven months, before her death in January 1999, Beth and The Lavender Trust contributed over £100,000 toward supporting younger women affected by breast cancer.

Following Beth's death, I was very proud to be invited by Jon to become a trustee of The Lavender Trust, which acts as the younger women's arm of Breast Cancer Care. Supported and sponsored by a large number of companies every year as their charity of choice, The Lavender Trust is as clear today in its mission to provide services and support for younger women affected by breast cancer as it was back in 1998. What a legacy!

Jane Tomlinson was another awesome example of a woman who, given a terminal cancer diagnosis, created an amazing legacy once she knew her time on earth was limited. Over the seven years she lived following her six-month prognosis, Jane not only created the most amazing memories for her children and her family, she undertook the most arduous of physical sporting challenges, pushing her cancer-ridden body ever further, and in the process raised almost £2 million for charity.

Although I never met Jane, I do know that the sense of urgency meant she pushed herself just that bit more, that bit further, to create her Post-Traumatic Success dream. As she got bolder and fitter, so the dream became bigger.

So I'm curious, how many people could *you* touch with your own Post-Traumatic Success dream? A handful? A few hundred perhaps?

I Dream a Big Hairy Scary Dream!

How many more people could you touch if you had a big, scary Post-Traumatic Success tarantula of a dream? What if you knew that whatever you put your mind to you could not fail? Just think, if you could help a few or even a few hundred people with your current goal, how many more could you help with a big, scary Post-Traumatic Success spider?

When I started out on my Post-Traumatic Success journey, I didn't know about the importance of defining a Post-Traumatic Success dream that was big and scary from the start, so mine has evolved over time from fairly comfortable, conservative ideas. In the early days of my own journey I wanted to help others going through the same traumatic journey of a breast cancer diagnosis.

In those early days of fundraising for Breast Cancer Care, shaking a tin outside Cavendish House in Cheltenham, I prided myself on being the most successful fundraiser outside London during October, which is Breast Cancer Awareness Month. One year I raised nearly £70 on a single Saturday (that was a lot of money back in the 1990s). I was pleased I was able to contribute and give back, proud of my success. However, I always had the niggling feeling 'this isn't enough'. In those days, £70 paid for the helpline to be able to run with three or four volunteers for about four hours; that was one shift, one of 11 shifts per week including Saturday mornings, 52 weeks a year. A drop in the ocean, in other words.

Standing with a collection tin outside an exclusive department store in an affluent part of the country wasn't scary; it wasn't a bit scary. It was hard work, for sure! If you've never held a fundraising tin or bucket for a charity, spare a thought for those who do; it's *really* hard on the shoulders and the lower back as the tin gets heavier and heavier! (It's especially hard when you know the weight is mainly small change and the odd foreign coin as people empty their purses, happy to be rid of the weight themselves!)

A plea on behalf of all charity fundraisers standing outside in all weathers for their worthy causes: pound notes or dollar bills are much lighter and easier to count!

So if it wasn't scary enough, what else could I do to 'up the scary stakes'? I was already helping out with the selection and training of new volunteers; as an experienced recruiter and trainer, that certainly wasn't scary!

What I hadn't really done up to that point was to talk with many women who were still *living* their traumatic event, women still in the grip of trauma. So I decided to join the 'front line' in Breast Cancer Care and apply for a weekly shift on the helpline.

Working as a volunteer helpliner gave me a vital insight into the huge differences there are in people's perceptions of the same thing. Some clients who called in to the helpline were distraught, having been told of their diagnosis *that day*; sometimes I was the first person they told, the first time they were saying the words 'I have breast cancer' to another human being. Other clients calling the helpline wanted some reassurance about a friend, or help in finding travel insurance or a support group after their diagnosis.

I remember my helpliner years as some of the happiest and funniest times of my life, which may seem an odd thing to say. Perhaps it was the extreme nature of the work we were doing there, with fairly rudimentary technical kit (even by 1990s standards), or maybe it was because I was allocated the shift with the most amazing bunch of women I could ever hope to spend time with. I like to think it was a mix of the two. I became a regular member of the Friday afternoon shift. We worked hard, we knuckled down when the phones were ringing, we laughed and cried with our callers, and I also remember laughing harder than I've ever laughed in my life when the phones were quiet.

You see, when you're in a small room with a bunch of women who have all known the trauma of breast cancer, and are working hard to help others going through the same, there are absolutely no taboos. None! Absolutely no subject is out of bounds. After all, we talked regularly with our callers about their most intimate fears and experiences. Often we were the only people they could turn to, to discuss sex during chemotherapy, undressing in front of their partner after a mastectomy or telling a new partner they've had breast cancer. We all had our own experiences of these events, and many of them entailed funny anecdotes that only another 'survivor' would understand.

My dear friend and one-time mentor within Breast Cancer Care was the hilarious Win Wyatt, who had been one of the founding members of Breast Cancer Care when it was called the Mastectomy Association back in 1973. Win was well into her seventies when I met her, and one of the most energetic septuagenarians I've ever met. Win could regale a room with her anecdotes for a month and never repeat a story. As well as her funny stories (like the one when the producers of *EastEnders* came to film the helpline for the Peggy Mitchell mastectomy storyline in 1999), Win had a unique way of making everyone feel comfortable in her presence. Her legacy will live on in the hundreds of women who attended her annual Strawberry Tea Party at her house in Catford, East London; the Strawberry Tea Party has become a perennial institution in the Breast Cancer Care fundraising calendar, with people holding them all over the country.

Win's legacy will also live on in the careers of the many hundreds of junior doctors, trainee surgeons and student nurses who attended her talks over the years. Often Win was the first breast cancer survivor they had met, and the only one, I'm sure, who regularly ended her talks by removing her blouse to give them their first 'full frontal' of her two mastectomy scars!

I joined the Breast Cancer Care helpline because I expected it to be a big, hairy, scary tarantula of a dream; I did not expect it to become the focus for fun in my week that it became. I genuinely spent all week looking forward to my Friday afternoons. Not that I didn't enjoy the rest of the week in my new-found self-employment; I did. But Fridays were special, they were my day of the week I spent with people who really understood me.

The helpline certainly didn't feel like the scary tarantula it was meant to be. I had to find a new tarantula!

Help: Tarantula Needed!

During this time I needed to stretch my comfort zone in a different direction. Speaking to people one-to-one as a peer supporter or on the helpline was becoming less and less scary, as things do when you've done them a few times. Breast Cancer Care's press department approached me and asked how I would feel talking to the press, telling my story as a motivation for others in a similar situation.

Being 32 at diagnosis made me different from most of my fellow breast cancer survivors, and being reasonably articulate with a good news story made me a popular target with journalists. Interviews with *Zest* magazine, *Woman & Home*, *Top Santé*, *Red*, *Woman's Realm* and *She*, as well as most of the national newspapers, followed, and again, these became less scary the more I did. An interview with Lorraine Kelly on Talk Radio was the highlight of that media-frenzied era; not only is Lorraine as friendly and easy to talk to off air as she appears, it was also a first for me to be live on national radio.

I'm Dreaming of a Post-Traumatic Success CREATION for You!

I'm guessing one of the reasons you're reading (and still reading) this book is that you're looking for some answers; some or all of the concepts in the book resonate with you and you're looking for a blueprint for creating your own Post-Traumatic Success. Well, you need look no further; it's time to work up your own Post-Traumatic Success CREATION.

There are a number of acronyms, often based on SMART, that are used, particularly in the corporate world, to help individuals and organizations set a direction for their plans and strategies. The problem with SMART objectives or goals is that while they work well for organizational goals where it is important to lay out a direction that is black or white, this is less helpful when it comes to our Post-Traumatic Success. Often Post-Traumatic Success is not linear or objective, it may be emergent and based on personal preferences, circumstances and subjective criteria. A Post-Traumatic Success CREATION, on the other hand, allows for shades of gray, different levels of granularity and changing circumstances.

CREATION stands for:

C – Clear and concise

R – Results-focused

E – Ecology-positive

A – Act as if

T – Team effort

I – Inspiring

O – Obstacle clearing

N – Next step

Let's look at these elements to your blueprint in more detail:

Clear and Concise

Have you ever set out to achieve something, only to realize that the plan you've made is too complex, too elaborate, and in fact you've set yourself up for failure? Setting a clear and concise direction for your Post-Traumatic Success means making it EASY to be successful, setting criteria for success that are easy to achieve. Oftentimes we make success such a difficult target to hit that we set ourselves up to fail, and will never have a sense of achievement, even if objectively we have created something special and of value to others.

What is it that would truly mean success for you? Is it writing a book? Raising money or awareness? If so, how much money? Is it working with a specific group of people? Finding a mate? Starting a family? Making your first $1 million? Creating a clear and concise blueprint makes it easy to focus on it, keep it front of mind and become aware of opportunities in that arena. Creating one that is muddled or overly complicated leads to distraction, displacement activity and often a feeling of overwhelm, and ultimately failure.

Results-focused

Stephen Covey said: "Begin with the end in mind." It's important to know what success will look, sound and feel like from the outset, so you will know it when it happens. As well as the tangible, the result of your Post-Traumatic Success will lead to an intangible feeling in you, and this is as important as the tangible result itself.

You may decide, for example, to write a book about your traumatic event. At one level, the result to be measured is the book itself. That alone, however, is an impersonal measure that is potentially soulless and empty. Where is the success in a book that no one buys, no one reads, no one engages with or reviews? Where is the success in a book that does not give the author a sense of pride, of achievement (or a corresponding bank balance) as a psychological or intangible result?

I know a number of people who, having focused on and achieved a tangible result such as a book, $1 million in the bank, or a challenging academic qualification have felt no sense of success or achievement inside. The tangible has not delivered the desired feeling. The results focus was single-faceted because the desired feeling was never established or expressed as a part of the desired result.

Ecology-positive

In the arena of NLP (neuro-linguistic programing) ecology has a specific meaning: it refers to the consequences now and in the future, for oneself and others, in various contexts such as home, career, lifestyle, as well as possible effects on the physical environment.

Your Post-Traumatic Success CREATION must be ecology-positive, meaning it will engender *more benefit* for you than you are *currently* enjoying, not only now but in the future. What does that mean?

Let's say a part of your Post-Traumatic Success journey involved giving up your job to start a business. Now, for most people, their first year in business will not necessarily be as lucrative, financially speaking, as their current salary. They need to find customers, build up their reputation and their goodwill in the marketplace, and they may well find themselves spending rather more than they bring back in as they pay to attend networking groups, buy raw materials, and have extra heating costs as they are spending more time at home now.

So how can this possibly be ecology-positive? The positives must outweigh the negatives to make it sustainable; in other words the benefits, even in the early days, must outweigh the costs. The benefit of no longer having to commute, sit in traffic day in day out, work in a bitchy office, be subjected to the manager's mood swings, put up with someone's cabbage diet permeating the office as the smell of stewed cabbage is spewed out of every air conditioning vent – you get the idea – outweighs the temporary drop in income and the sudden realization you can no longer call Fred in IT on extension 391 when your computer screen freezes.

Act As If...

In order for your Post-Traumatic Success CREATION to be successful, it's really important to *feel* successful from the start. One way to feel successful about something is to *act as if* it's already happening; talk about it in the present tense, celebrate even little milestones, hang out in the places successful people hang out, keep a journal for your learning and your successes along the way! In order to be more successful than those around you, you only need to be one step ahead.

As part of your acting *as if...*, why not find someone *you* can coach or mentor in your Post-Traumatic Success CREATION strategy? After all, as someone who has only recently progressed from where your coachee now stands, you are bound to have more empathy with his/her situation than the guru who is a hundred steps ahead and therefore less accessible. Stephen Covey suggests that teaching something within 24-48 hours of learning it yourself is a great way to deepen your own learning and create the 'muscle memory' you need to be *and feel* successful. This in turn could also help you to achieve the T, which is:

Team Effort

No man is an island; you do not have to travel alone along your Post-Traumatic Success path. The chances are there were lonely times when you were going through your traumatic event itself; even if you had fantastically supportive friends, relatives and counselors, I bet there were times in the wee small hours where you felt totally alone with your lot. Why, then, would you want to tread the path to Post-Traumatic Success alone?

Whether you find a coach to support and challenge you along the way, whether you barter time or services for the IT help you need, or whether you create a network of speed-dial friends, mentors and 'cajolers' around you to keep you on track, creating your 'dream team' is going to be vital to your being *and feeling* successful. Your dream team will be there for the bad hair days, they will also be there to celebrate with you; after all, who wants to celebrate alone? Someone once said to me celebrating alone is like eating a box of candy alone but with the wrappers still on!

Inspiring

I hope this criterion goes without saying... after all, if *you're* not inspired by your Post-Traumatic Success CREATION how can you expect to inspire others?

You have survived a terrible trauma, yes YOU, little ol' you! And now you want to draw the learning from that experience and turn the experience into something positive. If that's not inspiring, I don't know what is!

Your friends and family will be happy that you survived. The majority of people who go through what you went through will go back to the certainty of their pre-traumatic lives and pretend it never happened. And that's fine, I'm not talking to them. They're not reading this book. You are. So be inspired with your Post-Traumatic Success CREATION!

Do you want to know what the best thing is about being inspired by your own Post-Traumatic Success CREATION? You get to choose! You get to choose what it is, how inspiring you make it, when you get inspired by it, how much more inspiring you can make it... and all that in itself will inspire others to do the same. They'll take their lead from you; if you show up at your book launch, for example, at a 7/10 in terms of your inspiration, your audience will take their lead from you. At best they may make it to a 5/10 in their efforts to match you. Make sure your Post-Traumatic Success CREATION is inspiring for you; after all, you'll be living and breathing it for a long, long time, and you might as well be inspired by it. It will need to inspire you out of bed with a spring in your step even on those cold frosty mornings when all you'd really like to do is stay under a warm duvet. It will need to inspire you to turn off yet another mindless reality show on TV when the temptation to watch just another five minutes of brain-numbing drivel rears its particularly ugly head. You get the picture! Make it inspiring!

Obstacle-clearing

In those wee small hours, when you are sitting at an impasse with your Post-Traumatic Success CREATION and wondering why you ever thought this was a good idea, you may find your resolve dissipating. You may find doubts creeping into your mind, finding their way in despite your best efforts to remain inspired. There may be seeds of self-doubt, elements of feeling let down by others or by technology, thoughts of giving up and admitting defeat. Your Post-Traumatic Success CREATION must be big enough, strong enough and overwhelming enough to drive a horse and cart through these obstacles and keep you going no matter what.

We will talk in more detail about what some of those obstacles might be in Chapter 6.

Next Step

If you do not know what the next step is on the route to your Post-Traumatic Success CREATION, anything and everything is going to stop you getting started.

It's amazing how attractive that Everest-sized mountain of ironing looks, or cleaning out the kitchen cupboards (yes, even the one with the unidentifiable sticky stuff that got spilt ages ago in the back) when the next step isn't **clearly identifiable and easy**. Easy means something as straightforward as looking up the phone number of the person you want to interview for the book you might write, or coming up with five reasons why someone would NOT buy your knitted tea cozies when they're finished!

Here's the thing: if the thought of your Post-Traumatic Success CREATION is too big it will never get started. There will always be more important things to do first – always! It's like standing in front of a huge brick wall with PROBLEM written at the top of it. There's no way over it, it becomes demoralizing and disempowering. If you took that problem and laid it down on its side, with a few of the bricks set up as steps, and you stood on one of the steps, the next step would be clearly identifiable and visible. It's like standing on a chair to see what's on the shelf that's usually just above your eye level. Standing on a chair allows a completely new perspective on the kitchen cupboard – and life in general!

Exercise:
Your Post-Traumatic Success CREATION

It's time for you to create your own Post-Traumatic Success CREATION. I'd like to leave you the space to think about what's going to be important to you as you design it; take some time, perhaps with your eyes closed, thinking about what is possible, what you would like to happen, who you would like to work with and celebrate with, etc. You might want to think back to the first exercise you did in Chapter 1, where you designed your Oscar speech, or your Queen's Honours List speech. What has happened that has led you to your speech?

Now, what comes into your mind under each of the CREATION headings?

C – Clear and concise

R – Results-focused

E – Ecology-positive

A – Act as if

T – Team effort

I – Inspiring

O – Obstacle clearing

N – Next step

CHAPTER 4

"Hope in the beginning feels like such a violation of the loss,
and yet without it we couldn't survive."
Gail Caldwell, *Let's Take the Long Way Home:
A Memoir of Friendship*

The Buck Starts Here!

There's an old proverb that says 'The best time to plant a tree was 20 years ago; the second best time is now'. That's how I feel about your Post-Traumatic Success journey, and mine for that matter. Financial planners tell us the best time to start saving for our retirement is the time when most of us probably had other things on our minds than pensions – buying a car, going out on Saturday nights, and, let's face it, making ends meet financially.

At the time of going to press it was not possible for most of us to travel back in time, unless you had a hotline to Dr Who, so we have to make do with the second best time – now!

So there will never be a better time for you to start working on your Post-Traumatic Success CREATION than now, *especially* if there is an element of helping, serving or working with others involved. There are people out there absolutely desperate for what you have to offer; you'll have to trust me on that!

Waiting for the stars to be aligned, more money in your pocket, the recession to be over, the kids to leave home... these are all excuses. They are things you tell yourself to keep you from having to make changes; they ensure your certainty, they uphold the status quo for you. Except that they don't. You see, the fact that you're reading this book, and have read this far, tells me you're ready to embark on your Post-Traumatic Success journey, at least the next step. You're absolutely ready. It's your time, your time is NOW!

You Are Enough

I come across so many people who think they just need to go on one more course, read one more book, have a few more thousand dollars in the bank for a rainy day, or whatever the equivalent is, before they can get started. The important message in this chapter is you already have everything you need in order to start on your Post-Traumatic Success journey. If your dream for your Post-Traumatic Success involves starting something from scratch, something that will either make you more money or serve more people, or make you happier (or hopefully all three), why wait? Why defer your happiness, your financial freedom or your ability to help and serve others?

Whatever else it involves, your Post-Traumatic Success is about YOU, and it's about you right here, right now!

The only time that has reality is NOW; the past is nothing but a memory that has been constructed from a mix of events and our attitudes and beliefs about those events. The future is intangible, a vision, a hope or perhaps a fear. The only time that is concrete is right now.

So let's take stock of you, right now, in the present. What are your assets, what's your starting bid for your Post-Traumatic Success? If you've read any management books you've probably come across a SWOT analysis before, where you think about your:

S	*Strengths*: those things you can do, you have at your disposal or you have experienced
W	*Weaknesses*: those things you cannot do, do not feel confident about or do not have access to
O	*Opportunities*: resources, possibilities or people you can call on externally to you
T	*Threats*: people or things that could hinder you or stand between you and success

Exercise: SWOT Analysis

Go ahead, grab a coffee and spend 10-15 minutes just contemplating, and draw up a SWOT analysis for yourself as you see your current Strengths, Weaknesses, Opportunities and Threats.

Strengths	Weaknesses
Opportunities	Threats

Now I'd like you to take this a step further. You see, it's great to take what may feel like a clinical view of your strengths, citing skills you have, courses you've attended (qualifications you've attained) or work experience you've undergone in the past. And the weaknesses you've listed might be things you perceive others to have in greater abundance than you, be they skills, money, time, experience or other resources. I'd like you to go a little deeper now, concentrating on the here and now, concentrating on the person you see in the mirror, and really getting down to the basics of who YOU are and what you have available to you right now that will enable you to get on with your Post-Traumatic Success journey.

In fact I'd like to SHOWER you with success on your journey! The extra aspects I'd like to encourage you to think about are:

S | *State*: Carry out an audit of your current state when you stop and think about your Post-Traumatic Success journey. List the words that come to you, however contradictory they may seem; adjectives that describe your state or a state of X.

H | *Help needed*: If the help you need right now was abundant and you could call on whatever you need, what help do you need right now? This could be help with your Post-Traumatic Success CREATION or help that will free you up to get started: for example, childcare, someone to do the shopping or a sounding board for your ideas.

O | *Obvious*: What's staring you right in the face? What are you forgetting, or not realizing that you have on your side right now? Resources, willing people, a skill or personal attribute you hadn't thought about? And what else? And what else?

W | *WHY*: What is your big WHY for doing all of this? Are you creating a legacy for your children, following a long-held dream, carrying out a promise you made to yourself or someone else? Without a big WHY your motivation will ebb and flow as you get into your journey.

E | *Early success*: An early success, however insignificant, does wonders for the confidence levels and usually ensures the next milestone is much easier. What short-term success milestone could you set in place and celebrate as a morale booster along the way?

R | *Resources*: What do you *really* have at your disposal that you omitted in the SWOT exercise? Do your parents have start capital they could lend you? Do you have skills and attributes you didn't even count as they come so naturally to you?

Exercise: SHOWER Analysis

Now it's your turn again, and you know what to do. Coffee and thinking cap! You may find it beneficial to spend 10-15 minutes putting your initial thoughts together, then putting the paper away and going for a walk. When you come back to it an hour later, or even the next day, you're bound to come up with even more thoughts that your unconscious mind has filed away for you.

State	
Help needed	
Obvious	

WHY	
Early success	
Resources	

Job Description for Your Post-Traumatic Success

If you were to write the job description for the person who was going to create your Post-Traumatic Success successfully, what would that person need to be, do and have? Let's say Stephen Spielberg (or substitute a movie director of your choice) called you one day and said he'd heard about you and he'd like your permission to make the movie of your Post-Traumatic Success journey! After all, if it can happen to a bunch of Women's Institute women in Yorkshire who decided to raise a bit of money for charity by creating a calendar, or JK Rowling who wrote a children's fantasy story to make ends meet as a single mum, why not you? So who would play you? And what would they need to be, do and have to portray the real you in the movie? What attributes would they demonstrate?

Exercise: Post-Traumatic Success – The Movie

- *Who would play the role of you in the movie?*

- *Why?*

- *What attributes, qualities, skills and abilities would they demonstrate?*

- *How would you brief the lead actor? How would you direct them?*

- *Who would play the younger you in the flashbacks during the movie?*

I think the role of me in my life would need to be played by someone like Sarah Millican. I certainly don't consider myself to be an accomplished stand-up comedian and I don't speak with a Geordie accent, though I'm interested in dialects and I'd love to be able to emulate it. I do love her observational humor, her wry take on normal everyday activities and her tongue-in-cheek view of things she notices around her. She might have to work on her accent, though. With the best will in the world, I don't sound Geordie!

Knowing my luck, they'd probably choose Dustin Hofmann to play the role of me, and get him to dust down his women's clothes and reprise his role as Tootsie!

What does the job description need to contain; what would the successful applicant need to demonstrate to get the job of creating your Post-Traumatic Success? Writing skills? The ability to motivate and teach others? A wanderlust and an interest in other countries and cultures? Marketing expertise or the ability to network with people in power? The confidence to stand up in the *Dragon's Den* and pitch an idea that will make you a fortune or save the planet (or both)?

Exercise: Post-Traumatic Success – The Job Description

Write the job description for the role of creating your Post-Traumatic Success. What are the essential and desirable criteria for the role? What experience will the successful applicant need? Training? Skills?

Apart from the practical skills you may be thinking about, give some thought to the state the jobholder will need to be in as they embark on the Post-Traumatic Success journey.

Choose a Resourceful State

Why is this so important? Well, have you ever come across someone, perhaps at a party or a networking event, who tells you what they do or describes their business, but in such a low-energy, low-vibrational way you're left wondering how they ever get any customers? I've met coaches, trainers and even salespeople who, quite honestly, make me want to run for the exit! They might well be good at what they do, but the fact they don't seem to believe in their own product or service, or at least they give such a low-energy demonstration of their key attributes, I don't want to hear any more, and am certainly not motivated to sign up and pay money!

The first lawyer I met when looking for a divorce lawyer whom I could trust to represent my interests in court could not even make eye contact with me; she came across as half-hearted, nervous, unsure of the advice she was giving me, tentative in her answers to my questions... and I was the potential client! Heaven knows how quickly she might have crumbled when faced with an aggressive lawyer on the opposite side of the courtroom!

So what is a resourceful state? And what if I'm not feeling particularly resourceful?

Exercise: Let's Get Resourceful

Let's have a little fun with the first question: what is a resourceful state? How many different ones can you come up with? Here's a start:

• Happy	• Healthy
• Can do attitude	• Lucky
• Curious	• Energetic
• Analyzing	• Reflective
• Abundant	• Knowledgeable
• Wealthy	•
•	•
•	•
•	•
•	•
•	•

What state would you like to be in, in order to 'meet your public'? To a certain extent this will depend on what your public is expecting of you, what is needed for the particular stage of your Post-Traumatic Success journey, and to a lesser extent on what the situation demands.

When I started working on the Breast Cancer Care helpline on Friday afternoons, I could not answer the phone with my usual Tigger-like bounce and energetic voice tone until I knew who the caller was and what they were calling for. Someone who has had a diagnosis this morning is not ready for high-energy bounciness, they may well need someone who can empathize, and show understanding by syncing with the speed of their speech and breathing. They will probably want someone who will walk alongside them for a while, metaphorically at least, as they get used to the implications and gravity of their situation.

If your Post-Traumatic Success journey is likely to involve supporting and serving others through counseling, coaching, or teaching, for example, it is paramount that you take the time to get yourself into the most resourceful state possible so you can model this for your audiences. A coach can have all the technical skills and qualifications possible, but if he or she cannot get himself/herself into a state with energy, conviction, trust, self-belief, confidence, strong resolve or whatever is called for and expected by the client, he/she will be a hungry coach!

Similarly, if your Post-Traumatic Success dream is to travel the world, you had better conjure up a state of curiosity, tolerance of difference, and resilience in the face of new experiences before you board the airplane!

Controlled or Controller in Your Life?

What if you're not feeling very resourceful when you need to, for example if you're meeting a journalist to be interviewed, or you're writing an article on your experiences? In Chapter 2 I talked about a body of research that has been carried out by a number of management thinkers, notably by John Rotter and more recently, Suzanne Kobasa, on a concept called the 'Locus of Control'. There are some people who believe firmly that the locus of control resides within them, and that they alone have the power to choose how they feel, choose their state in any given

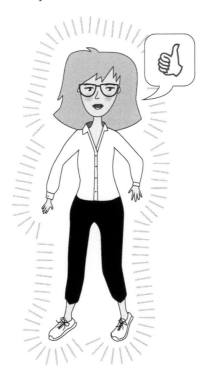

situation, and choose the meaning they attribute to an event. Such people are therefore able to access a whole range of states in an instant. So the question now becomes, 'How do I become a person with an internal locus of control?'

One of the first (of many, many hundreds) of lessons I learned from Tony Robbins, the Grand Master of resourceful states, was this:

Change your strategy =>
change your result

Change your story =>
change your life

Change your state =>
you change it all!

If you are in an unresourceful state, perhaps your energy is low, you're tired and lethargic and you're finding it hard to motivate yourself, here are three things you can do to change this in an instant:

a. Change Your FOCUS

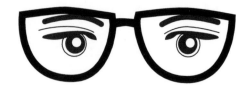

If you've been staring at a computer screen for ages, or concentrating on a problem, a negative comment from someone or a situation that's pulling you down, you can literally change where you focus. In a physical sense this might mean getting up and looking at something else for a while: your Dreamboard, for example, or a picture of your family or pet – something that has the power to make you think and feel differently. Give yourself a few minutes away from the energy sapper, physically focusing on something positive, and notice how this changes the way you think and feel about the problem. Could you have a sign above your desk with a motivational quote, a joke or cartoon, or just the word 'Success', for example?

b. Change Your LANGUAGE

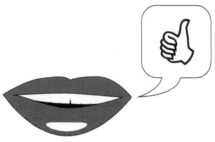

What words and phrases have you been using, either to describe a problem or person, or even internally with yourself? Have you caught yourself giving YOU a hard time, being mean or uncharitable when something didn't work out as you wanted? What if, just for five minutes, the problem went from being a major catastrophe to 'a minor inconvenience'? How could that change your state and help you to find a more resourceful one?

Take the words you used to describe the person (especially if that person is you!) or problem and say them with a Donald Duck voice. How about setting them to music – the theme tune to the *Dambusters*, for example, or the *William Tell* Overture?

c. Change Your PHYSIOLOGY

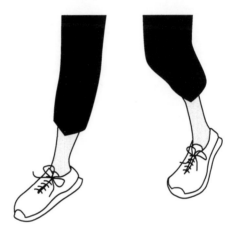

Get up and move around – literally move the energy. How quickly can your mood change if you get outside in the fresh air, go for a walk in the park – or just move into the kitchen to make a cup of tea? If you have the chance for greater movement, things always seem less drastic after some exercise; in my younger days I played squash regularly (rather more enthusiastically than skillfully!). I can't tell you how many faces I've managed to visualize in that little green ball in my time! If they only knew!

The point with these changes is that if you're the sort of person who tends to feel the locus of control lies externally, with someone else, God, the Universe, your ex or whoever, these are practical things you can do very quickly to change your situation. If you don't always find it easy to control (choose) how you feel about something or someone, change something else that you *can* change – your focus, language or physiology and look with interest at what else changes as you do that.

Making sure you embark upon your Post-Traumatic Success journey in a resourceful state will ensure success with ease, success that you can enjoy along the way, rather than feeling things are a constant struggle. A more resourceful state is likely to lead to success more quickly than a less resourceful one.

Think about it: if you're in a state of feeling stressed, uncertain, under-confident, angry, resentful, overwhelmed, tired etc. about the project you're creating, how might that impact on decisions you make, how keen you are to work on the project, the vibes you might radiate to others when talking about it? How easy would it be in an unresourceful state to attract or recruit others to *want* to work with you, support you or even listen to your ideas? I'm sure you have had experience in the past of being around 'energy vampires' or 'drains', people who can't or don't want to summon up the resourcefulness they need for themselves, and end up draining it from those of us who have more than enough to go around.

Richard Wilkins, self-appointed Minister for Inspiration, talks about our 'script', in other words the thousands upon thousands of lines, stage notes, cues, rules and directions that are handed down from our parents, grandparents, teachers and carers from a very young age. For many of us, the script may act as a restrictor, holding us back from the choices we might otherwise make, or the things we might otherwise do or say differently. Richard asks the question: "Which would you choose?" Would you choose the script that has taught you over many years that 'life is hard', 'success comes to those who work hard', or even 'people like me don't deserve success'? If it were down to you, would you really choose to be one of those people who inhabits the planet purely to make others feel or appear more successful? Really? Would you choose to be one of the also-rans?

Surely no one in their most resourceful state would choose to believe these things? If that were the case, how would life's successful people know that was what they were put on the planet for, while the rest of us somehow knew our place? What would give them that knowledge, that they were the 'chosen' ones?

The answer has to be linked to how resourceful they feel, surely? After all, is it true that the most successful people you meet (however we define successful) are always better looking, better qualified, better experienced or more intelligent than us? I know that isn't true for me. In a resourceful state I know I can give many who are more qualified, more experienced and much more beautiful a run for their money. The difference comes back to where I feel or believe the control to be in that moment. Is it within me, or is someone else holding on to it?

For me it's almost always inside me. Even if I can't choose to change the situation itself, I can *always* choose how I feel about it. By changing something about me, my focus, language or physiology, something over which I most certainly *do* have complete control, I do get to choose, and I get to change the situation – namely my relationship to it.

Exercise: What Would You Choose?

Your turn now! What would you choose to do, think, feel, see, hear, believe or even disbelieve, if the choice were entirely yours? Spend a little time just enjoying your own company, perhaps with a pen and paper to hand. The following questions are intended to open up your thinking / feeling, not limit or restrict you in any way. As ever, some will resonate more than others.

If you could choose your state, your *most* resourceful state:

* *Who would you choose to spend time with?*

* *What would you choose to feel?*

* *How would you choose to spend your days?*

* *How would you choose to feel – about yourself, your situation, your Post-Traumatic Success?*

- *How successful would you choose to feel?*

- *How would you choose to communicate – with yourself, with others, with your higher self?*

- *What would you choose to think?*

- *What risks would you dare to take?*

- *Who would you choose to model?*

- *Who would you choose to be?*

When you choose to create something in a resourceful state, there's more chance you'll actually enjoy the journey.

In Chapter 5 we will explore how you make sure you surround yourself with the people who will help you do this.

CHAPTER 5

"The test we must set for ourselves is not to march alone but to march in such a way that others will wish to join us."
Hubert Humphrey

Surround Yourself with your SUPREME Team

You may be feeling out of your comfort zone by now – either a little outside it, or indeed way, WAY outside it and into the next zip code! After all, we've talked about big scary spiders, we've considered what it means to give up on 'normal' (does that automatically make us abnormal, then?) and in the last chapter I suggested ignoring everything your parents taught you and choosing your own resourceful path...

Well, I'm hoping in this chapter you'll get to relax a little, as you realize that you're not expected to do it all alone. In fact I'd go a step further and say "thou shalt not go it alone!" If you're going to enjoy the journey and breathe life into your Post-Traumatic Success CREATION, it would be pretty dull and boring, not to say lonely and more than a bit scary, if you were to do the whole thing alone.

No, this chapter is all about creating the ideal team of people around you that I'd like you to think of as your SUPREME Team. Your SUPREME Team will consist of the people you will need for moral support and motivation, the people who will pick you up when things don't go your way, and the people who will be there to eat cake with you when there's something to celebrate. They may also be the people you need around you to cajole, bully or even 'guilt' you into staying on your path when those self-doubt gremlins start creeping in to question your judgment.

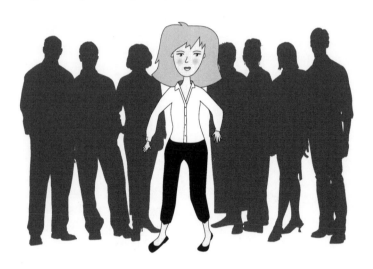

What is a SUPREME Team?

Chances are there will have been times during the traumatic event you went through when you felt very alone, even lonely, as you worked through the stages of the trauma. You may have felt at times as though you were the only one experiencing your trauma, that no one else could understand what you were going through, or no one else was able to help.

As well as the motivation and moral support you will gain, your SUPREME Team will consist of members who can help with practical, tangible things – like getting your laptop or tablet to work when it gives up at the most inopportune moment, or sorting out bits of technology that won't speak to each other. You may wish to find the ideal person who will cook dinner for you when you've worked through the day and haven't stopped to eat all day! This chapter will help you to identify the people you need in your SUPREME Team, and help you with practical hints and tips on how to recruit, repay and retain them, even if you're just starting out.

A SUPREME Team differs from the friends and family who were there to see you through the traumatic event itself. While there may be some crossover, a SUPREME Team should not be confused with those people who were there out of loyalty, friendship or a sense of family duty to see you through a crisis. You will probably find the majority of friends and family members will want things to go back to 'normal' after the crisis itself as that will feed their need for certainty.

If your Post-Traumatic Success journey is to take a different route, those who need the certainty of returning to the way things used to be pre-trauma will not cope with being members of your SUPREME Team. They may try to warn you off your plans and hold you back. For those looking for certainty or wanting to return to 'the way things were', your Post-Traumatic Success journey will be too uncomfortable, too different, too uncertain. It threatens the status quo, and thus their certainty.

Your SUPREME Team will consist of a number of roles, some of which may be filled by the same person, others might be quite distinct and therefore need a specialist. Some of the roles might be paid, others voluntary or offered on a bartering basis. You may even have two or more occupants for some of the roles, and some roles may be time-limited as your Post-Traumatic Success journey progresses.

The attributes you need to recruit into your SUPREME Team are:

S | *Supportive* – You need SUPREME Team members who are on your side, who will be there to cheer you on, pick you up, advocate for you and, if necessary, remind you why you are following your Post-Traumatic Success path and be your own personal cheerleaders.

U | *Understanding* – Members of the SUPREME Team must have a clear understanding and appreciation of your Post-Traumatic Success CREATION, and its importance in your journey, so they can best support you in its implementation. They must understand the impact on you and others of *not* following your Post-Traumatic Success path.

P | ***Party-loving*** – Celebration is an important part of your Post-Traumatic Success journey, so have someone on the team who ensures that successes large and small are celebrated along the way. You will want your SUPREME Team to celebrate with you as this will be hugely motivating when the journey becomes rocky along the way.

R | ***Responsibility-focused*** – One of the jobs of your SUPREME Team is to act as your conscience and hold you responsible or accountable for the actions you have planned to take; they might call into question any behaviors or activities that seem to take you further from your Post-Traumatic Success journey.

E | ***Enabling*** – You will want SUPREME Team members with a 'can do' attitude, members who will look for ways to make things happen. They may have the necessary contacts themselves, but if not they will look for ways to make things possible. They will not accept defeat or fall at the first hurdle.

M | ***Mentors*** – Do you know someone who is ahead of you on the path you would like to take on your Post-Traumatic Success journey? Is there someone with the skills or experience you need who would be happy to join the SUPREME Team and stretch you to your chosen CREATION?

E | *Expertise* – By surrounding yourself with others who have some specialist knowledge that will help your Post-Traumatic Success, you will be able to shorten the journey, short-circuit your learning and arrive at your destination sooner. Recruit people into your SUPREME Team who have supplementary skills, or an interest in picking up the necessary tasks you don't want to focus on.

How to Create a SUPREME Team for Free

Now, not everyone's Post-Traumatic Success CREATION is going to generate the large cash sums that would be necessary to build an army of well-paid experts and specialists around you. By this stage you might be thinking *it's all right for you to talk about SUPREME Teams, I don't have that sort of money.*

It is probably true to say that the majority of us will not be in a position to start recruiting a team of salaried staff around us as we start out on our Post-Traumatic Success journey. After all, if you have recently lost your job, undergone treatment for serious illness or perhaps suffered a relationship break-up or even a bereavement, you are probably not going to be feeling particularly flush with cash. In fact the traumatic event itself may have left you struggling financially.

So where do you find the right people with these skills and attributes for little or no cost?

Well, the answer may be easier than you think. In the UK we have a huge network of organizations that are set up with the sole purpose of helping others through specific traumatic events. This network is far bigger, more dedicated and much better resourced than in many other countries I know; from established charities and networking groups to informal local self-help groups, there will be an interested group of people focused on your agenda.

Now, while the charity *per se* may not be what you are looking for, the chances are that someone working within that organization, either as a salaried staff member or as a volunteer, will be on their own Post-Traumatic Success journey, and may be just who you need to recruit.

Alongside the physical networks of people you may find who are on a similar Post-Traumatic Success journey of their own, we of course also have access to worldwide networks of potential SUPREME Team members through online forums, interest groups, chat rooms, etc. You do not need to look very hard on the internet to find websites, blogs, online meetings of others who share your interests or are on a similar journey. You can get *free* support, advice, even funding these days, without leaving the comfort of your armchair.

Exercise: Create Your SUPREME Team

OK, let's get specific. Let's think a little closer to home.

There are three steps to this exercise:

Step 1

Close your eyes and imagine your Post-Traumatic Success CREATION as it grows, takes on a form, a life, a soul; imagine your journey as you wake up each morning and plan what you will do today to bring your Post-Traumatic Success CREATION a little closer to fruition. Now think about who is accompanying you on that journey:

♥   Who is there, by your side, celebrating every success, every breakthrough with you?

♥   Who is there smoothing the path for you, removing obstacles and sorting out issues that might trip you up?

♥   Who is your wingman, your Girl Friday? Perhaps you have more than one of those people as you go through the different stages of your Post-Traumatic Success CREATION, from its conception through the different milestones in its growth.

♥   Who is spurring you on, on the rainy days of your journey?

♥   How are the different members of your SUPREME Team interacting with each other? How are they demonstrating their love and dedication to you and your journey, every day? How are they supporting and complementing each other?

♥   How are they holding you accountable to yourself and your Post-Traumatic Success?

♥   How many SUPREME Team members are there? Do you recognize them all, or do you have new members who have joined because they believe in what you are doing?

♥   What are they saying – to you, to each other, to third parties?

♥   When they speak about you, how do they speak? Describe the voice tone, the language they use.

...

Step 2

Take a piece of paper and create either a mind map or a table with three columns. On the page, quickly write a list in the first column (or as separate legs of the mind map) of all the people you can remember who were present in your meditation in *Step 1*. Write their names and/or the roles they undertook in the meditation of your SUPREME Team. Make sure you leave space so you can add to it as other SUPREME Team members come to mind. At this stage there is no maximum number of SUPREME Team members.

Next to each name, write down a few words to describe what qualifies them to be in the SUPREME Team. What personal attributes or formal qualifications do they possess? Some of your SUPREME Team members may be as yet nameless people, identified by their skill or personal attribute alone: for example 'an accountant', 'a fitness instructor' or 'a Facebook specialist'. That's fine, too.

Step 3

This is where you think about what you may have to offer each SUPREME Team member that is not necessarily money. Where can you barter something you have for something you would like from them? Some examples may be:

- ♥ Swapping childcare, i.e. alternating play dates that buys you time one afternoon a week in exchange for feeding your child's friend on another, and saves on organized childcare that can become expensive and is often inflexible. I have several friends whose entire childcare is based on this model, week in week out.

- ♥ An hour a week's book-keeping in exchange for a new website.

- ♥ Buying an hour a week of cleaning in exchange for some exam tutoring for their teenager (only if you can create economies of scale by tutoring several at once for different SUPREME Team members, or combine it with tutoring your own kids, for example).

♥ Ask your employer for a more flexible working arrangement – a combination of longer and shorter days, for
example. Does your employer offer sabbaticals for
long service? Might they, if you were to put forward a
mutually beneficial proposal?

♥ Consider asking your ex for a more flexible access
arrangement that allows you larger blocks of time for
attending workshops or writing your book. This has
worked very well for me in recent years to the extent
that I have managed to carve out more Post-Traumatic
Success time than I would have done if we'd still been
married. This does presuppose a positive and mutually
respectful relationship with your ex, something which,
in my case, has been a gradual, if not always smooth
process, developed over many years. Some longer
standing members of my own SUPREME Team can
attest to this!

♥ Ask your ideal SUPREME Team marketing guru to
teach you some of his/her techniques in exchange for
testimonials, home-cooked meals, a banner ad on your
website, produce from your garden, a joint venture or
lessons in a skill you possess.

♥ What about enlisting the help of your children? Even
very young ones will step up to the challenge of
helping out, especially if they know they are helping
toward a bigger purpose. A lot of fun can be had
changing their own duvet covers, putting laundry away,

> setting the table, etc,, while they're too small to be designing websites, leafleting the neighbors or editing your promotional videos. Believe me, that time comes sooner than you think! The currency for my own kids progressed from a comic in the early days, as a thank you for a job well done, to a trip to Starbucks while out shopping (the free Baby Chinos, an espresso cup of milk froth you get when you buy an adult drink, were always a hit).
>
> ♥   ...

I have many friends and clients who have successfully bartered all of the above, plus much, much more. All it takes is a little creative thought and a healthy dose of self-confidence, combined with a pinch of courage. Oh, and be prepared to be amazed at some of the results you might achieve.

One friend arranged for her neighbor's au pair to clean her house one morning a week in exchange for an hour of conversational English over a cup of tea. Another, whose Post-Traumatic Success CREATION was to start a charity following the birth of her child with profound special needs, grew her self-confidence and her courage by creating her ideal SUPREME Team around the needs of the fledgling charity. She was inundated with offers of time, computer skills, marketing campaigns, even office space and laptop computers. In exchange she offered a year's free membership to the charity.

Who Needs a SUPREME Team?

The answer is 'everyone does' – even you!

I hope you're convinced that no one can, or indeed *wants to* plan, organize, implement and celebrate alone. Where's the fun in that? No one wants to have to motivate himself/herself to carry on when the going gets tough, and chances are no one is going to have the skills, abilities and motivation to carry out all the tasks involved in your Post-Traumatic Success CREATION. Your SUPREME Team, however, will be *your* hand-picked selection of people with the necessary attributes to ensure that *your* Post-Traumatic Success dream becomes a shiny, sparkly reality.

And who wants to celebrate alone when everything starts falling into place, and you start seeing the fruits of your efforts? Do you really want to be eating candy all alone with the wrappers still on? Make sure you have the right SUPREME Team around you to celebrate with you!

Whatever you desire for your Post-Traumatic Success, you *will* need to find people who are more skilled, experienced or just more motivated in certain aspects of it than you are. Whether your Post-Traumatic Success CREATION is writing and publishing your memoires, raising money for a worthy cause, traveling the world and broadening your horizons, or following your dream career, you will need the help of others. Teachers, mentors, marketing experts, trusted advisors, travel guides, experienced fundraisers, accountants, perhaps also a cleaner, gardener or help with childcare might be on your list of job roles that will be needed. I hope the exercise enabled you to identify these people and also to become more aware of the skills, experience and attributes that *you* possess, for which others would be truly grateful.

I had been planning this book in my head for the best part of 20 years before I got down to writing the first words. So what was it that stopped me actually putting pen to paper during that time? It wasn't a lack of writing skills, as I train my corporate clients to write business reports, sales proposals, marketing brochures and even the patient notes for prescription medication. It wasn't even really a question of time, as I have no more time now than I did 10 years ago; I still have access to the customary seven days in every week, 24 hours in every day, 60 minutes in every hour, just like you or anyone else.

What has made the difference has been creating my SUPREME Team around me. From Mindy, my book coach, who is keeping me focused on the goal and the process, to the au pair who ensures I can ring-fence the concentrated writing periods needed to move the word count forward, my SUPREME Team is made up of specialists who carry out their specialism, thus ensuring I can shut myself away and write. From Helen who ensures the worst of the dust in my house is cleaned once a fortnight, to Maurice who stops the proportion of weeds to planned plants from reaching pandemic levels in the garden, I can focus on the things that really make me happy, fulfilled, and ultimately on finding creative ways of being able to pay them to do what they do.

Does that mean that without my SUPREME Team I could not have written the book? Well, not exactly. I *am* capable of cleaning my house and pulling up weeds in the garden; however, neither of these things is a task I particularly enjoy. To be honest, if I needed to find the time to do these things now, I would procrastinate, prevaricate, protract, and find all the displacement activities under the sun *not* to do these tasks.

In terms of bartering, I set up an arrangement with my two children a few years ago which works very well. Being a busy single mum who is constantly juggling a business, charity work, Mum's taxi service and homework, while trying to ensure we have healthy balanced meals, I have always been an advocate of making sure my children understand the balance between work and earned rewards. As a result, they now have their regular jobs to do around the house (emptying the dishwasher, garbage and compost bin, hanging up the laundry and changing their own bedding), for which they earn their pocket money. For extra jobs there is extra reward, which may be monetary or may be negotiated – extra time for play before bedtime, for example.

I have included an extra clause into the contract with my children: they earn their pocket money for carrying out their jobs *without complaining*. They rue the day they signed up to that particular clause!

My children are, after all, star members of my SU-PREME Team; they are supportive, understanding, party-loving, responsibility-focused, enabling in their attitude, even mentors on occasion, and in some aspects also experts.

Leader of the SUPREME Team

All teams have a team leader or a team captain, be they work teams in the corporate world, or sports/recreational teams. Your SUPREME Team is no different, it needs a leader who is resourceful, confident, motivated and the sort of person the Team is willing and ready to follow.

As your SUPREME Team's leader, your job is to provide the leadership and direction which makes them want to follow you.

What does this mean for you?

It means you need to work out what sort of SUPREME Team leader you want to be, and work at being that leader.

What do you associate with the term 'leader'? Giving instructions? Knowing everything better than the team? Being in charge? Disciplining poor work performance?

Well, all of these things may be true to a certain extent; however, there are other attributes that are said to mark leaders out from the pack, be they in the workplace or in the playground. You see, leadership is not confined to the corporate boardroom; look in any playground and you will see immediately who the leaders are, and who, by definition, are the followers. In the playground it might be the child actually skipping while the others dutifully swing the rope. In the boardroom it could be the person who manages to stop all disputes and mini conversations in the room with a look, a hand gesture or a facial expression, without uttering a tone.

There are certain criteria that are shared by all leaders, irrespective of whom or where they lead; I'd like to share a selection of these with you here. I have spent many years studying management skills in organizations, and learning what it takes to be a good manager. These skills tend to be quite tangible and measurable, whereas I have found in the course of my corporate training work that leadership skills are harder to identify in a consistent way, and by the same token harder to capture using language that means something. As with many things, it is sometimes easier to start with what non-leaders *don't* have or do; this might help identify what differentiates the few who are real leaders.

1. *Leaders have followers – if no one is following you, you're not a leader!*

   It's perhaps too obvious to say that in order to be a leader, you *have* to have followers. If I may make a polite suggestion: take a look behind you right now – do you see anyone following you? Is there anyone listening to you, agreeing with you, believing in you and supporting what you say? Without followers it's hard to get leverage or traction for your ideas; you might be seen by others as different, lacking in credibility, a crackpot even, and if there's no one refuting that on your behalf, those negative messages might be louder than yours.

2. Leaders show their vulnerability – if you're afraid to show ALL of you, you're living a lie

Some feel it is dangerous or weak to admit they're vulnerable, they're learning or they're human after all. What are they afraid of? Being exposed as a human being? Being shown to have flaws, just like others? Who has more credibility as a leader of people for you: the super-human, robotic, 'perfect' untouchable or the person who has walked your path, who has had real experience of pain, anxiety or uncertainty and has come through it stronger and more determined to learn from it?

3. Leaders pick their SUPREME Team and nurture/ develop them – if you're doing everything yourself you're a lone wolf (or a control freak!)

Do you think Richard Branson, Oprah Winfrey, or Jamie Oliver with his campaign for healthier school meals, build their own websites, design their own logos or even come up with all of the ideas that have put them at the forefront of their game themselves? Of course not! They have gone out and found the experts in their own fields and brought together the SUPREME Team that together can build much better results than any one team member in isolation. Leaders spend time and effort nurturing that team, creating the environment to motivate them to **stay together.**

4. *Leaders feel the fear and do it anyway – if you're allowing fear to stand in your way, acknowledge it, thank it, move on!*

   Fear can paralyze us at the most inopportune moments: when we need to move out of danger's way, when we see a great opportunity whose impact could be life-changing, or when we stand before a breakthrough in our personal development, for example. For some, the process of acknowledging the fear and acting anyway comes quite naturally. Others need to learn a process to do this, and go through the process steps almost manually:

   - Recognize the fear has come up to keep you safe

   - Acknowledge it (ignoring it is impossible anyway)

   - Thank it – after all, its only function is to keep you safe

   - Click the override button and move on

   - Choose a more resourceful thought to replace it – you on a podium with a 1st Prize rosette, for example, or sitting on a beach enjoying the fruits of your efforts

5. *Leaders strike out and try new things – if you're swimming with the flow, you're a follower just pretending to lead!*

Take off the trainer wheels and go! They cause drag and pull you back. If you're swimming along with everyone else, they will use your 'slipstream' to catch you up and eventually overtake you, as the elite runner overtakes the pace-setter on the approach to the finish line. Leaders look at what everyone else is doing, and make up their own mind. After all, we'd still be working on the assumption the world was flat and that human beings would explode if they traveled faster than 30mph!

6. *Leaders are naturally more resilient – if you're feeling lethargic or unmotivated, choose a more resourceful state*

    Leaders have bad moments, even bad days from time to time. Many have experienced seriously traumatic events in their lives; the difference is they don't stay there and allow these to become the pattern. They understand that they are not their trauma, it is but a part of their make-up. Instead they look for the learning, take the opportunity to do something about it, make changes and come back stronger as a result.

7. *Leaders surround themselves with others who are better than they are in key areas – if you're afraid to be shown up by your SUPREME Team, you probably are already!*

    Just like the advertisement for bathroom cleaner, there is always someone who loves to do the jobs you hate! So let them! Ask yourself the question: What is the best use of my time right now? Or, if

I were going to add $100, $1,000 or $10,000 worth of value to this endeavor this morning/this week, where do I need to focus my effort? It probably isn't standing behind your web designer asking inane questions and holding her up from her work!

8. *Leaders find creative ways around obstacles – if you allow obstacles to stop, disable or divert you from your Post-Traumatic Success course, they will eat away at your self-esteem*

What if you looked upon obstacles as your friends, playing a prank on you to test your resolve? This is, after all, your Post-Traumatic Success journey! By its very nature it is different from the path you have trodden in the past – as with any uncharted territory, there are bound to be tests, challenges, even huge great boulders along the way. You are there to draw up the map for those who come after you!

Some obstacles can be blown out the way using brute force, others will need to be persuaded, cajoled and coerced to move. Others still will need to be circumvented by creating a kink in the path to get around them. In sailing this is known as tacking; the shortest distance between two points is a straight line, except when it isn't! If the wind is coming from the direction you wish to sail in, you have to sail at an angle of around 45 degrees to the left, then 45 degrees to the right to get around the obstacle called the wind.

Once you have your SUPREME Team in place, you will be better equipped to deal with the obstacles that will line your route. Chapter 6 will help you recognize those obstacles for what they are, and help you to get over, through or around them.

CHAPTER 6

"A lonely day is God's way of saying that he wants
to spend some quality time with you."
Criss Jami

Get Out of Your Own Way

However committed you are to following your
Post-Traumatic Success path, chances are that not everything will run entirely smoothly on your journey
to success. Whether tangible or intangible, whether
founded in reality or not, there are going to be obstacles, challenges, hindrances and wobbles that will test
your resolve and tempt you to doubt yourself.

'But my obstacles are real' I hear you say. 'I *really* don't
have any money for marketing' or 'I *really* have been
knocked back by 50 publishers'. These statements may
appear true, and therefore may present themselves as
trip-steps to someone with less resolve and resourcefulness than you.

But you? You have come through a traumatic event
in your life, an event where you had to summon up a
lifetime's worth of courage, resourcefulness and energy to put one foot in front of the other and keep going
on days when that must have seemed a tall order. Are
you really going to be beaten by an everyday, run-of-

the-mill bend in the road that, let's face it, at the height of your trauma would have seemed a minor inconvenience by comparison?

Once again, it comes down to choices. We make choices constantly throughout the day, most of them without thinking. When we come up against a fork in the road, particularly one we were not expecting, or one that presses certain hot-buttons within us, certain things happen within our brain and our physiology that may cause us to doubt what we thought was true.

Use Your Brain for a Change

In order to understand better how these challenges or forks in the road might present themselves, it is worth taking a bit of time to understand the human brain, and how the different sections of it function. I'm sure you are already aware that the brain is made up of different areas, each of which has a different function in keeping this body of yours alive and safe. Let's just remind ourselves what happens when we are growing our comfort zone, stretching the pantie elastic and stepping into the unknown.

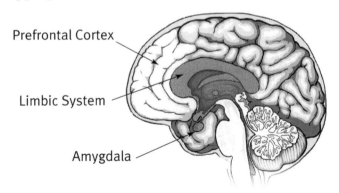

Prefrontal cortex

This part of the brain is involved in planning; it is responsible for complex cognitive behavior, personality expression, decision making, and moderating social behavior. Also included in its list of tasks are: abstract thought processes, problem solving, creative thought, reflection and co-ordination of movements. It is sometimes called the 'executive' for the brain; its basic activity is thought to be the orchestration of thoughts and actions in accordance with internal goals.

When you set yourself a goal to lose weight, quit smoking or raise $10,000 for charity, this is your prefrontal cortex working at its best. New Year's resolutions are decided, planned and committed to in this part of your brain.

Limbic System

The limbic part of the brain is responsible for all our value judgments, emotions and feelings. Picking up on non-verbal cues and communication is done by this part of your brain and, as we know, these are a much more genuine and believable language than the persuasive words that may have been crafted and created by the prefrontal cortex.

Whether we wish to believe it or not, our emotions are the key drivers in decision making, in fact we will run a decision through the logical decision-making filters only to rationalize or justify an emotional decision that has already been made.

Consider this: you have set a goal (or announced a New Year's resolution) to lose X pounds in weight. You've planned how you will do this, how you will balance a reduced calorie intake with more exercise, you've filled in the application form for the gym and you've been shopping for the ingredients for your new eating regime.

Now, on Monday you plan to go straight to the gym after work, then go straight home (without stopping for the usual latte with friends, and without swinging by the takeaway shop on the corner). Just before you finish work, you get a call from a good friend who is distraught; her idiot of a boyfriend has left her again and she's just discovered she's pregnant. She's desperate, she has no one else she can turn to, you're her best friend, she can't do this on her own... (I'm paraphrasing, you get the idea).

I double-dare you to tell me you would make your apologies, explaining that today of all days is the day you'd planned to start your new fitness regime... if she'd called any other day... There's no decision to be made, is there? The friend wins every time. The point is, not only do our emotions make most of the decisions, they make them without conscious thought or deliberation, and they tend to hit us with the immediacy and power of a direct order – unconsidered, unannounced, and more often than not impossible to resist.

Of course I played on the emotions very specifically in that example; if that was too obvious, and you're still not convinced, consider these situations:

- You decide to get up early tomorrow morning to go for a run before the rest of the family wakes up. Your child (or the dog/cat) picks this night of all nights to wake at regular intervals and need your presence (or the neighbor decides to throw an all-night party), so you finally get to sleep an hour before the alarm is due to go off.

- You set aside a few hours on Saturday, your only free day of the week, to work on your book as you have agreed a specific word count with your book coach by Monday. Saturday comes and you wake up with a headache/your mother calls and asks if you could run her to the supermarket as her car won't start/a long-lost friend calls/the family see you working at your desk and assume you are fair game for untold disruptions.

- You proudly post your first blog and ask a couple of trusted friends to read it and comment as you plan for this to become a regular feature. Their comments are hesitant, lukewarm or non-existent.

- You're on Day 3 of your new diet and fitness regime, which involves eating certain foods and avoiding others. You discover you've missed the bus home, the next is in an hour, so it will be rather late by the time you get home and have prepared your healthy meal. You're really hungry now. You happen to find candy in your bag.

- You have spent a lot of time putting together the copy for your new webinar series which you plan to launch next month. You receive an email from a well-known speaker on the circuit in your sector, with an invitation to sign up for his webinar series on exactly the same subject – for half the price you were planning to charge.

- You weigh yourself after the first week of eating more consciously and healthily, to find you have not lost a single pound.

I could go on with these examples. Some will resonate with you more than others. The point is, our best-laid prefrontal cortex plans can very easily and quickly be challenged, questioned, or completely scuppered by the limbic system, whose job it is to fire emotional torpedoes as if to remind us who's boss!

Amygdala

Within the limbic brain, the amygdala is the first part of the brain to actually receive the emotional information. It acts as the alarm system for the brain, taking in all the external stimuli (physical, psychological, emotional) and making instantaneous decisions on whether or not it is a threat. It processes emotions such as fear, anger and pleasure, and is responsible for laying down the memories that are stored in the brain.

Conditions such as anxiety, autism, depression, post-traumatic stress disorder, and phobias are suspected of being linked to abnormal functioning of the amygdala, often caused by damage, developmental problems, or neurotransmitter imbalance.

So why does all of this matter? I hear you ask. After all, you didn't find this book in the Biology GCSE reference section of the book store, did you?

Well, it matters if we are going to discover what may get in the way of your Post-Traumatic Success and stop it from happening. There are a number of things that tend to show up as real, tangible obstacles designed to take us off course from our Post-Traumatic Success path, which we can deal with once we understand them and know why they are showing up.

Let's look at the main 'banana skins' on the route to success in more detail; after all, if we can summon up the courage to look the enemy in the whites of the eyes, maybe we can acknowledge it, then out-stare it and make it disappear.

Fear of Failure

This is probably one of the biggest reasons people have for not starting, or at least stopping short of experiencing real success. And yet if we read the scientific journals, we know that the only two fears we come into the world with are the fear of being dropped and the fear of loud noises. So where does the fear of failure come from? What is it that we *actually* fear?

One thing that differentiates human beings from the rest of the animal kingdom is the ability to imagine. We are able to imagine all sorts of things: what it might feel like to win the lottery, the humiliation of making a mistake in front of hundreds of people on a public stage, the feeling of holding your baby for the first time, etc. Even those of you who profess to be more logical than creative have imagination.

In fact I would go so far as to say anyone with children (or a special person in their life) has the ability to imagine. Picture this scene: it's a school night. Your son/daughter was supposed to be home at 10pm and it's now 10.45pm. The last bus is long gone, they're not answering their cell phone, you haven't managed to reach any of their friends by phone, text, Facebook or carrier pigeon.

What are you imagining right now? Add to this the fact that the last conversation you had with him/her was an argument about homework, or you hear the traffic information on the radio and there has been a serious accident near your house. Perhaps you're watching *Crimewatch* on TV.

I don't need to continue. I'll assume I've convinced you of your very advanced and abundant talent in the arena of imagination!

The trouble with our imagination is that our subconscious mind is so gullible it's unable to tell the difference between imagination and reality. The scenario I painted above is not real, it's made up. And yet if you do have children of the age where this could conceivably happen, you might well find yourself developing the same symptoms you would if you were trapped in a cage with a hungry lion. Once again I have to rely on my imagination for that one!

The thoughts, feelings, emotions and even the physiological responses would have been the same if you had *actually* received a phone call from the police or hospital – excessive sweating, raised blood pressure, blood draining from the head, muddled thinking, etc. Why is that? Well, the simplest answer is that the mind and body are one organism, so whatever is going on in the mind will be passed on and replicated in the body. That happens in our subconscious, without even having to think about it. That's why horror movies, romantic love movies, cop dramas, etc. work so well. We get the physical and psychological feelings as if we were on the set.

So here's the problem: while we tend to be very good at linking the hypothetical to our responses when it's negative (some more than others), many of us seem to stall that mind-body connection when it's positive. We seem to unlearn that connection as a rite of passage into adulthood. I'm sure we all remember the anticipation we felt in the lead-up to a celebration – Christmas if you celebrated it, or your birthday, for example. Even the eagerly anticipated arrival of a friend for a playdate used to be a source of great excitement in those heady pre-cell phone days. These days, my own children seem to spend the entire build-up phase texting back and forth, so the anticipation is lost.

Why, then, don't we spend more time imagining how good something could be in the future, and enjoy the feelings, symptoms and sensations now? Well, many people do – through visualization exercises, manifestations, vision boards, gratitude diaries, for example. What a pity we have to relearn such techniques as adults!

Fear feels uncomfortable, uncertain, unsafe, and many choose instead to stay comfortable, certain and safe. The most basic human need in Tony Robbins' model of the world is the need for certainty, and most people we meet in life will gravitate toward that their whole life through. Those people, generally speaking, do not tend to pick up a book like this, so I congratulate you on getting this far along your path to Post-Traumatic Success!

I have one quick question for you before we move on: who defines failure? Who defines whether you succeed or fail at something in your life? Something like, say, starting a business, or writing a book? You do, don't you? So if you're writing the rules, why not make it easy to succeed? And hard (or impossible) to fail?

Sometimes we can be our own worst enemy when it comes to defining success and failure for our ventures and our lives. I sometimes ask my clients: "How would you know if you had been successful in X?" You would be amazed at how complicated some people make it to feel successful:

♥   My book would need to be an Amazon bestseller within three weeks of publishing *and* I would need to be offered a publishing deal on the back of it

♥   My business would need to turn over six figures within the first year *and* be nominated for a business-of-the-year award

♥   X would have to write me a letter with an unreserved apology for the hurt he has caused me and my family *and* show his remorse by paying me $10,000 in compensation

♥   I would need 100 unsolicited testimonials for my work from people who didn't know me before

♥   I would need to lose 40 pounds by Christmas (it's November now!) without increasing my exercise regime

♥   I would need to run my first marathon in under three and a half hours *and* look as fresh as a daisy at the end

And so on. Sometimes people combine two or three rules, all of which need to be achieved in order to feel successful. Failure, on the other hand, is often much easier to attain:

•   I feel fat after eating a cake ☹

•   I didn't lose seven pounds on that crash diet this week ☹

•   No one smiles when I board the subway train ☹

•   I *don't* find $10 on the sidewalk ☹

•   I don't win the lottery ☹

•   My boyfriend doesn't propose to me ☹

•   My boss doesn't praise me for the report that took ages to write ☹

With rules like this, everybody can be successful at something, namely failing!

Need to be Perfect

Perfectionism is a myth, it doesn't exist except as a concept in our heads. There, I've said it now. What is the definition of a perfectionist?

'Perfectionists strain compulsively and unceasingly toward **unobtainable** goals, and measure their self-worth by productivity and accomplishment. Pressuring oneself to achieve **unrealistic** goals inevitably sets the person up for disappointment. Perfectionists tend to be harsh critics of themselves when they fail to meet their standards.' (Wikipedia)

'... displeased with anything that is not perfect or does not meet extremely high standards.'

So there we have it: perfectionism is unobtainable and unrealistic, and it therefore sets us up to fail from the start.

Needing to be perfect is an interesting concept in itself, and it begs the question: Where does this need (or 'straining') come from? It probably originates for most of us from a time in the past when we really wanted to do something well, and feel proud of our efforts: that essay at school, the thank-you letter to a grandparent, our lines in the school play. The problem arises when something happens, someone says something to dash that pride. The essay has a spelling mistake, we fluff the lines in the play slightly – whatever our hopes for the perfect performance, we have come up short, we have not lived up to the exceedingly high expectations we had of ourselves, or we assume others had of us.

The need to be perfect will paralyze you into inaction; for fear of not being perfect, you may be tempted not to start at all, or not to publicize your work, or to apologize unnecessarily. The phrase 'imperfect action not perfect inaction' is very appropriate here!

I'll Be Ready When...

The psychology behind deferring success is an interesting one, and probably for many of us harks back to a time in childhood where our parents told us we must work hard before we can play. Eat our vegetables before we can have any dessert. We can't have happiness, riches, success, fun, etc. until we have done something to deserve it. This leads many people to defer these things until they believe they have deserved them.

I have worked with clients who felt they needed to defer their success for all sorts of reasons; here are some favorites:

- My children are young, I should wait to start my business until they're older

- I don't have a financial cushion yet, I can't leave my job till I've saved a bit more money

- I just need to learn a bit more/go on one more course before I can start coaching others

- I'll wait till I'm a bit more confident before I learn to drive

The reality is, if this is holding you back, there will probably never be a right time to start on your Post-Traumatic Success journey. You will learn along the way and be able to incorporate the learning as you go along. After all, a baby doesn't wait until it's done all the courses and read all the manuals on learning to walk before it pulls itself up on the furniture and has a go. In fact I bet a baby doesn't even realize that it's not an expert at walking when it first tries it out! No one told him/her that they weren't very good at it; as a result, they keep on trying, incorporating the feedback from their environment as they go.

So I wonder – what would need to happen for you to enjoy the journey toward your Post-Traumatic Success, rather than deferring it to a time when some pretty tall hurdles have been overcome? What would need to happen for you to just get started and have a go?

Need to be Liked

It probably goes without saying that most of us want to be liked by others. Why, then, do we allow this excuse to hold us back, to keep us from trying out new things? In reality most people would not actually recognize this phenomenon in themselves, and yet when it comes down to it, they stay safe, thus keeping those around them feeling safe.

The reality is the human species does not go looking for change, as a rule. We are creatures of habit, we like predictability in our lives, we like to know what to expect in certain situations, and we derive a certain comfort from the status quo. This is, of course, more true for some than for others. You and I both know the exceptions to this rule: people who have made radical changes in their lives, gone to live in a different country or changed career, life partner, hair color, political leaning, even gender, to name a few examples. Generally speaking, as humans we only go looking for change when the status quo becomes untenable, uncomfortable, or perhaps too safe, and where the alternative looks more attractive and the cost of moving there seems surmountable.

The Formula for Change was created by Richard Beckhard and David Gleicher, and is usually referred to in management training as the Gleicher Model of Change.

$$D \times V \times F \dashrightarrow R$$

Three factors must be present for meaningful and lasting change to take place. These factors are:

$D =$ Dissatisfaction with how things are now

$V =$ Vision of what is possible

$F =$ First concrete steps that can be taken toward the vision

If the product of these three factors is greater than

$R =$ Resistance

then change is possible. Because D, V, and F are multiplied, if any one factor is absent or low, then the product will be low and therefore not capable of overcoming the internal resistance to change.

If the resistance comes from the possibility of hurting others, making others feel uncomfortable, creating bad feeling, upsetting a relationship apple cart or becoming unpopular as a result of the proposed change, this may stop the change happening or being sustained in the face of the resistance. If the resistance comes from one's life partner, social or faith circle, or from the fear of being 'different', the change may not happen, or it may be started but may be reversed at the first sign of an obstacle – real or perceived.

The classic situation, which you may have experienced personally, is attending a personal development seminar, conference or workshop and leaving after a day or two fired up, motivated and determined to implement the new learning. What happens when you leave the sanctity of the back-slapping, supportive and high-octane arena of the training program, carefully clutching your exquisitely crafted and very ambitious action plan and a fistful of business cards, and return home to an expectant family, partner or co-worker? Do they welcome you home with open arms and demand that you teach them every nuance, every nugget, every distinction from the weekend immediately, before putting the kettle on or opening the wine bottle? Do they heck!

The more likely scenario is that your absence has been more noticeable by the fact that the refrigerator is now empty (as no one has been shopping), the house looks like a war zone, and you very quickly end up feeling somehow guilty for having been away at all. Rather than enthusing your nearest and dearest with the strategy you have for transforming the family's/business's fortunes, you end up tucking away your now less-than-shiny action plan, playing down just how much fun you've had around such inspiring people, and time-traveling right back to status quo-land, to a time before the training where you felt controlled by circumstances and in control of nothing.

How do I seem to know so much about this? Well, I'll just have to leave you guessing on that one!

Fear of Success

There is a widely accepted phenomenon within personal development circles: who you hang out with is who you become. Think about the five or so people you spend most time around. As you think about them, what do you notice about their personal financial situations, their incomes, their levels of health and fitness, their values, etc? If you were to add up the incomes of the five people and divide by five, this is likely to be close to your own income level.

Let's suppose this is true for you; how do you feel about this, as you think about these people? Obviously they are your friends and family, you are not choosing to follow your Post-Traumatic Success dream in order to turn your back on them. And yet the fact that you are choosing to plow a different furrow, to stretch the pantie elastic in some way, may well come across like this.

How will you manage your existing relationships while creating space in your life for the new ones, the people who are sharing your Post-Traumatic Success path, at least for now? How could it be possible to nurture both? How could it be possible to segment or compartmentalize your friends, at least until the existing friends start to see and encourage the changes in you?

The reason these questions are often so hard to answer is that our fear of success can actually be greater than our fear of failure. This sounds like an odd thing to say, especially in a book entitled *Post-Traumatic Success*. I know, hear me out!

Think about a time you saw someone speak at a conference or had a conversation with someone about something spectacular they had achieved – perhaps they had written a book, run a marathon, raised a significant amount for charity or manifested their dream job. Maybe that person spoke about how much easier the achievement had been than they had expected. I wonder what your little voice inside your head said at that point... Was it 'Wow, that sounds great, I bet I could do something like that, I must ask her for some tips'? Or was it more like 'That's all well and good for her, she had lots of help, an army of childcarers, cooks, trainers and PR gurus to help'?

If you're anything like me, I suspect the latter was closer to the truth. Why is that? Well, believe it or not, that little voice in our head has our best interests at heart, and everything it says is intended to keep us safe. Yes, really!

How does putting me down and making me feel small keep me safe? I hear you ask. Well, it keeps us safe from the fear we have that if we were to become bigger, better, richer, slimmer, more famous, etc. than our peers, we might lose them.

Tony Robbins' model of the six basic human needs demonstrates the balancing act between our need for significance and our need for connection with others. There is a balancing act between the two because too much of one can lead to a loss of the other. If I have a high need for or crave connection and affiliation with others, I will do nothing to upset the apple cart, or stand out from the crowd. I will do everything I can to fit in, even if that means subconsciously subordinating my own dreams and desires in favor of the collective.

Think about it: what do children in the playground say to the child who does better than the rest in a class test, or shows up with the latest trainers/pop cult CD before the rest? 'Class swot', 'Show-off', 'Too big for her boots', etc.

How many people do you know who spend their lives self-sabotaging, keeping themselves small, fitting in, often just at the point where their dream could come true?

The reality is we try so hard to fit in, when really we were put on the earth to stand out, to be a glittering star, to use our attributes, skills and our *differences* to step away from the crowd and shine our light in front of everyone, rather than hiding it under the proverbial bushel. The reality is we are too fearful of the consequences of success beyond our dreams, rather than the opposite.

It's time to redress that balance between our need for connection with others and the significance of shining our light for the *benefit* of ourselves and others. How big could your Post-Traumatic Success dream really be if you stopped playing small and shone your light into the world instead?

Exercise: What Stops You?

Time now to take a step back and consider what some of the trip-steps or obstacles might be that have stopped you shining your light up to now. There is a series of questions in this exercise under each of the headings. Some will resonate with you more than others. As you read the questions, sit and think about each one for a few seconds, and allow your subconscious mind to really sit with it and immerse itself. You may not come up with lots of answers straight away, but your subconscious mind will continue to consider each one long after you have moved on to the next chapter.

Fear of Failure

* *What does failure look, sound, smell, taste and feel like for you?*

- *What would mean that you had failed?*

- *What would the impact be of failing? On you? Your family? Your business? Others?*

- *What else?*

- *And what else?*

- *What would others say if you failed?*

- *How would you know you had failed?*

- *What are your references for failure? Parents? Other significant influences on your life?*

- *What happens to people who fail?*

- *Where else have you personally experienced failure? What happened?*

- *Where else have others experienced failure, where you disagreed?*

- *Can anything good ever come out of failure?*

- *...*

Need to be Perfect

- *What does 'perfect' look, sound, smell, taste and feel like?*

- *How do you know when something is perfect?*

- *What would mean that you were imperfect?*

- *What is the impact of not being perfect? On you? Your family? Your business? Others?*

- *What else?*

- *And what else?*

- *What does it mean to be 'not perfect'?*

- *What would others say if you weren't perfect?*

- *What are your references for imperfection? Parents? Other significant influences on your life?*

- *What happens to people/things that are not perfect?*

- *How do you deal with other people who are not perfect?*

- *Can anything good ever come out of something not being perfect?*

- *...*

I'll Be Ready When...

- *What does 'ready' look, sound, smell, taste and feel like for you?*

- *How do you know when someone is ready?*

- *What would mean that you were ready?*

- *What's the impact of not being ready? On you? Your family? Your business? Others?*

- *What else?*

- *And what else?*

- *What would others say if you weren't ready?*

- *What does it mean to be 'not ready'?*

- *What happens to people/things that are not ready?*

- *Can anything good ever come out of not being ready?*

- *...*

Need to be Liked

- *What does 'liked' look, sound, smell, taste and feel like for you?*

- *How do you know when someone is liked?*

- *What would mean that you were liked?*

- *What's the impact of not being liked? On you? Your family? Your business? Others?*

- *What else?*

- *And what else?*

- *What would others say if you weren't liked?*

- *What does it mean to be 'not liked'?*

- *What happens to people/things that are not liked?*

- *Can anything good ever come out of not being liked?*

- *...*

Fear of Success

- *What does 'success' look, sound, smell, taste and feel like for you?*

- *How do you know when someone is successful?*

- *What would mean that you were successful?*

- *What's the impact of being a success? On you? Your family? Your business? Others?*

- *What else?*

- *And what else?*

- *What would others say if you were a success?*

- *What does it mean to be a success?*

- *What happens to people/things that are a success?*

- *Can anything good ever come out of being a success?*

- *...*

Not Having a Big Enough WHY

Why do we do anything in life? Why do you get out of bed every morning, go to work, make the choices you make? We all *think* we know the reasons we do things, but how often do you actually take a step back and ask yourself the question?

Some of us will say: "I'm working three jobs to pay the bills" or "I do this to provide a good role model for my children." These are all very commendable things, but if fear is still getting in the way of your Post-Traumatic Success dream, your WHY is not big enough. Your big WHY which will make your Post Traumatic Success dream a reality.

When it came to writing this book, my fears stood in the way for too many years. One day during 2013, my 20th year since my big traumatic event, I finally decided my WHY was bigger than all of those fears put together.

CHAPTER 7

"Do not wait and hope to be discovered…
make yourself so you cannot be denied!"
Jamie McCall, *Living the High Life Without Drinking the Champagne*

Your Step-by-Step Action Plan to Post-Traumatic Success

Well, we're almost there! This is the last chapter in the journey to get you started on your Post-Traumatic Success dream. I hope you're as excited as I am for you, and eager to get started! This chapter is about getting your action plan together so you will have no reasons at all to procrastinate or be uncertain. By the end of this chapter you will have everything you need to make a start, including clarity about your vital first step.

The hardest part of any change or project you may be embarking upon is taking the first step. Once that first step has been taken, all further steps become relatively easy by comparison. Until you take the first step and have therefore embarked, you have not really committed fully, you could still back out, delay, procrastinate, find excuses and not 'fail'. In some people's model of the world, you can only fail at something if you actually take action.

I would venture a step further; the most stressful, worrying or anxious time is actually the moments immediately before you take the first step: going on stage, speaking in front of a large group, pressing 'send' on an expensive purchase online or saying 'yes, go ahead' to the tattoo artist. I have experience of all but the last one!

Why should this be? Well, taking the first step means *committing to change*, to something new. By definition, the first step means it is something new, something unknown. I remember the feeling clearly the day I went in to have my breast cancer operation: January 11, 1994. Life had been building up to this for what seemed like half a lifetime; in fact it was 11 days. By the day of my operation I was almost climbing the walls by my fingernails with the anxiety.

Sometimes the first step seems too onerous to take, and this might stop us for years and years.

This chapter holds the ultimate process steps for you to begin on your Post-Traumatic Success journey; it will provide you with a step-by-step guide to ensure you never again become paralyzed at the first step. This is a process which I follow myself when embarking on a new project, and if for some reason I try to take a short cut, I always find myself backtracking and going back to square one.

There are three steps to your Action Plan:

Step 1: Gratitude – Enjoy the Future *Now*

I am sure we are all aware of the need to thank people who help us in our day-to-day life *after* the event, and you may already practice gratitude on a larger scale for events in the past as a daily practice too. I keep a Gratitude Journal which I write in regularly; as well as writing down my gratitude for the people, things and events I already have in my life, I also practice gratitude in advance for the things that I *wish* into my life – before they actually appear. Sometimes I go a step further and get positively excited about future events, as if they had already happened. Enjoy the future now – that way, if it does happen you get to enjoy it twice, and if not, well at least you got to enjoy it for a while.

If you're not used to doing this, the concept is going to sound very strange, frankly perhaps even certifiable. After all, weren't we told as children: 'Don't get too excited, it may not happen'? My friend and mentor, Richard Wilkins of the Ministry for Inspiration, will tell you that's exactly why we should get excited. Our physiology can't tell the difference between a thought or feeling and the real thing. After all, most of us are very good, some might say even expert, at the strategy of worrying about something in the future before it actually happens. Don't believe me? What happens when you watch a horror movie, a love story or a movie where a cute little fluffy creature is injured or dies? What happens inside your head, what happens to your blood pressure, your body temperature, the muscles in your shoulders, your tear ducts… need I go on?

So why not use a strategy that we already know works, and merely change the actors' cues and the subtitles?

This exercise is a little different but works along the same lines. Stephen Covey, who during his life was a management consultant, speaker and author of *The Seven Habits of Highly Effective People,* suggested we should 'begin with the end in mind'. In fact this is his Habit Number Two. He takes the concept of the 'end' to extremes, as he invites the reader to attend their own funeral and imagine what others might be saying about them. This metaphor doesn't really sit well with the whole concept of Post-Traumatic Success, so I'd like to propose a much more positive exercise.

Exercise: Begin With the End in Mind

This is your opportunity to really start enjoying the future before it happens! I'd like you to experience how it's going to be when you've followed your Post-Traumatic Success Action Plan, and you are now enjoying the fruits of your success.

Part 1

You can close your eyes for the start of this exercise if that helps you create pictures and video sequences in your mind's eye. Imagine you've been busy creating your Post-Traumatic Success for a while now. You have had some great moments, your SUPREME Team has really stepped up for you, and you are now at an awards ceremony to celebrate your success. It could be a ceremony like the Oscars, a specific industry sector or charity accolade, perhaps even the Queen's New Year's Honours List. Wherever you are, it is a momentous and a joyous occasion; everyone who means anything to you is there to watch you receive your award. Think about these questions as you picture yourself there, receiving your award for all your effort and your success:

- *Who is there with you?*

- *Who do you need to thank?*

- *What did they do to help you to this point today?*

- *Who is going to be handing you the award?*

- *What have you achieved that is being recognized today?*

- *What else?*

- *And what else?*

- *Where have you come from? What was your start point?*

- *How long has it taken you to get to this point?*

- *What were the milestones along the way?*

- *What obstacles have you smashed through or removed to get this far?*

- *What was your big WHY? Why was achieving this so important to you?*

- *What would the consequence have been of not achieving this?*

- *Who else will benefit from your Post-Traumatic Success dream today?*

- ...

Part 2

So now you've enjoyed all the people who are there watching you receive your award, celebrating, clapping, enjoying the moment with you. Now as you receive the award into your hands, you find yourself pulling your carefully planned acceptance speech out of your pocket. What does it say? Who do you need to thank?

What have you written in your acceptance speech? Please write it down here, so you have the words, the sentences and everything you want to say written down here in front of you.

You may wish to write it on a clean sheet of paper so you can attach it to the wall in front of your computer, or leave it lying prominently near where you tend to work.

How was this exercise? Were you able to conjure up a little excitement, energy and enthusiasm for your Post-Traumatic Success dream before it actually happens? I hope so.

Step 2: Your Purpose

If you're thinking this next step sounds a bit pink and fluffy, I would invite you to suspend judgment and do the exercise. This step is an absolutely vital planning tool, and apart from the fact that I have used it to help thousands of my corporate clients to plan their reports, client proposals, presentations and new projects over the years, it is a step I undertake myself at the start of anything new. I really practice what I preach.

The process is so simple as to be insulting to one's intelligence, yet profoundly powerful. It involves sitting and thinking, and coming up with all the questions to which you need answers, before you can start. Importantly, it involves not leaping straight into the need to look or feel busy, and start producing the final document at the planning stage. It is a step to be undertaken *before* putting pen to paper or fingers to keyboard.

We'll give the process some structure to make it easier.

The problem for many people is that once they have an idea, they want to get started immediately with 'doing', and will often throw themselves into activity or 'busy-ness' without stopping to think. Busy-ness is at best a displacement activity, at worst an energy-sapping, confidence-robbing distraction, and dangerous to the survival of our Post-Traumatic Success.

Getting busy is a bit like building a house by starting to build a wall; in your haste to get busy, you start laying bricks on top of each other and mortaring them together without knowing where the wall is going to go. Trouble is, you can't decide where the wall should go once it's built; from the little I know about house-building, you're supposed to build the wall in situ, i.e. where it is actually going to go. Ideally with some foundations first!

The Purpose stage comes even before the foundations – this is the architect's planning stage. It's called the 5WH stage.

The six most important question words in the English language are:

Who, What, Why, When, Where and How.

In fact, they are so important Rudyard Kipling wrote this poem about them in 1902:

I Keep Six Honest Serving-Men

I keep six honest serving-men
(They taught me all I knew);
Their names are What and Why and When
And How and Where and Who.
I send them over land and sea,
I send them east and west;
But after they have worked for me,
I give them all a rest.

I let them rest from nine till five,
For I am busy then,
As well as breakfast, lunch, and tea,
For they are hungry men.
But different folk have different views;

I know a person small –
She keeps ten million serving-men,
Who get no rest at all!

She sends 'em abroad on her own affairs,
From the second she opens her eyes –
One million Hows, two million Wheres,
And seven million Whys!

Exercise: Who, What, Why, Where, When, How

We're going to make this so simple it will really feel as though I'm insulting your intelligence. I make no apology for that – the simpler the better at this stage. And I have no interest in massaging your ego; that won't get your Post-Traumatic Success dream implemented!

The idea is to come up with as many questions as you can that begin with the open question words Who, What, Why, When, Where and How. These are questions to which you need the answers, or at least to have considered possible answers before you can move on. Let your questioning mind flow; write down as many questions as you can – at this stage it doesn't matter if they seem relevant or not. The great thing is your subconscious mind will really run with these questions, and start 'googling' through your internal filing cabinets for answers. So don't judge, justify, sanitize or rationalize, just allow your creative juices to flow.

I've come up with a few questions under each of these question words to get you started.

The more questions you have, the more they will help you identify and spec out your Action Plan for your Post-Traumatic Success. There will be almost limitless questions beginning with each of these serving-men questions, and they will help you really focus your Action Plan and make its implementation much easier. Once you have answers to the questions, you can discard anything that is not Post-Traumatic Success-shaped. You can stay on track and dismiss any distracting thoughts, confidence-robbing gremlins or interruptions masquerading as good ideas!

Who

- *Who is in your SUPREME Team?*

- *Who do you need to deal with or work with to implement your Post-Traumatic Success?*

- *Who could hinder you in your path?*

- *Whose permission do you need?*

- *Who has a vested interest?*

- *Who is your competition in achieving this?*

- *Who is going to LOVE it?*

- *Who is your biggest fan?*

- *Who knows your audience better than you do?*

- *Who...?*

- *Who...?*

- *Who...?*

What

- *What resources do you need?*

- *What's the worst case scenario?*

- *What are you offering?*

- *What do you want to achieve with this?*

- *What are they expecting?*

- *What do they want/need from you?*

- *What else could be possible?*

- *What if you knew you couldn't fail?*

- *What if...?*

- *What's the BEST thing about your Post-Traumatic Success dream?*

- *What are you most looking forward to?*

- *What would you like to delegate?*

- *What can you do to make this even more fun right now?*

- *What would make you ecstatic right now?*

- *What...?*

- *What...?*

- *What...?*

Why

- *Why is this so important to you? And to others?*

- *Why now?*

- *Why is this an absolute MUST for you?*

- *Why should they listen?*

- *Why will they follow you?*

- *Why will you carry on, even in the face of obstacles?*

- *Why not do something far more interesting instead?*

- *Why...?*

- *Why...?*

- *Why...?*

When

- *When is it going to start?*

- *When will you know you've been successful?*

- *When will you celebrate the first milestone?*

- *When will it be okay to announce your success?*

- *When will it be okay to dance around the table?*

- *When...?*

- *When...?*

- *When...?*

Where

- *Where are your SUPREME Team right now?*

- *Where are you in your planning?*

- *Where is your greatest excitement around your Post-Traumatic Success dream?*

- *Where do you get your resourcefulness from, even on rainy days?*

- *Where can you go for help or support?*

- *Where are we now?*

- *Where in your body will you feel the success?*

- *Where...?*

- *Where...?*

- *Where...?*

How

- *How will you feel when your Post-Traumatic Success Dream comes to fruition?*

- *How will you celebrate the milestones?*

- *How do you want others to feel?*

- *How are they feeling right now?*

- *How will you know you've been successful?*

- *How are you feeling right now?*

- *How could you choose a better state right now? An even better state?*

- *How will you fill yourself up?*

- *How could it be possible?*

- *How...?*

- *How...?*

- *How...?*

There are two main reasons for asking all these questions at the outset, before embarking on your Post-Traumatic Success adventure:

1. *Audience* – If your Post-Traumatic Success dream involves others, for example contributors to your charity, sponsors for your event or attendees to your workshop, who is your audience? What do you need to know about them? What makes them a homogeneous group?

2. *Purpose* – It's really important that you know your purpose when it comes to your Post-Traumatic Success dream; what is the end in mind to which this should lead? Think back to your 'Oscar Speech' at the start of this chapter. What are you receiving the award for? What are people saying about you? How have you changed their lives for the better or inspired them to make changes themselves? What have you done that has perhaps impressed, surprised or entertained them? Can you complete this sentence?

... in order to...   so that...

For example:

I have written this book **in order to** inspire other women who have experienced trauma in their lives to choose a resourceful state **so that** they may also discover their Post-Traumatic Success dream.

I want to raise $100,000 for cancer charities **in order to** fund vital support and care **so that** younger women affected by breast cancer need never feel alone with their illness.

I want to travel across Australia and New Zealand **in order to** better understand how other cultures live and work **so that** I can embrace my love of traveling, broaden my horizons and write a book about my experiences.

What you really need to do is spend some time gathering all your thoughts, plans, information, visions, desires and wishes together in one place, in order to start distilling your Post-Traumatic Success plans. Take it from me, investing the time to do a good job at this stage will save you time, irritation, blood pressure and possibly money as well. I know what I'm talking about!

You see, **Step 2** serves one vital purpose for your Post-Traumatic Success dream, and that is to save you from *OSINTOT*: **O**h **S**ugar, **I N**ever **T**hought **O**f **T**hat!

I always find if I start something without the vital *OSINTOT* step, I invariably take longer to get going, I make mistakes, I go back and correct stuff, I start trying to be all things to all people – and ultimately I end up putting my need for 'busy-ness' on hold and coming back to this stage. And invariably there were all sorts of things I hadn't thought of.

Step 3: The Architectural Design

There are a number of ways you can go about this stage in your Action Plan. What you really need as an outcome here is a blueprint to take forward to the next stage, so you know exactly what you need to do, and where, when, how, etc. One of the biggest reasons for procrastination is not having a clear enough plan at the architectural design stage, with a clear and *easy* first step. Take it from one who knows, if the first step is not easy, the rest of the plan could be written on toilet paper and archived away in a vault somewhere, for all the good it will do.

So what does this mean, an easy first step? Imagine you were standing in front of a very high fence, or better still a brick wall. There seems to be no way over, under or around it. It's just a big wall with Problem written on it. This is your Post-Traumatic Success project, at least while you are standing before it. Imagine, on the other hand, the brick wall broken down into its constituent bricks. The bricks are formed in steps, so all you need to do is climb on to the first step. From there you will see on to the next step and so each step is visible once you have climbed the previous one.

How easy is it now to climb over or around the wall?

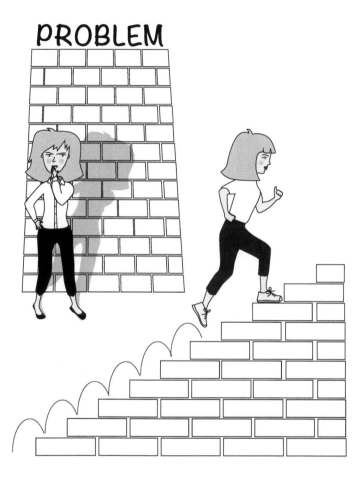

An easy first step might be to find phone numbers for three fitness instructors in your area in order to ask them to quote for a number of personal training sessions. It might be to spend 20 minutes researching websites for charities that help people with dyslexia, evening classes in your area in Swahili or local business coaches who offer a trial first session to new entrepreneurs.

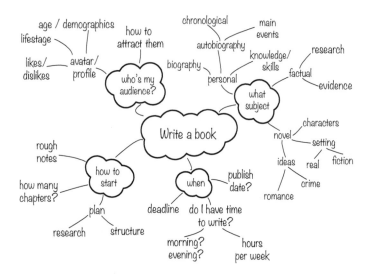

The way I create my Architectural Plan is using a mind map or pattern note. For more information on mind maps, seek out any of Tony Buzan's books on the subject. I find the use of spatial awareness works very well for me, and I am able to create a flow around the map which gives me a structure, while at the same time making my Action Plan very visual and easy to add to and follow. Some people work well with flowcharts, Excel spreadsheets or Microsoft Project, for example. A list in Microsoft Word or a pad of A3 paper and some colored pens will work just as well if you're a beginner at this. Please don't allow yourself to become distracted by the method for capturing information for your Post-Traumatic Success Action Plan; it would be a shame to allow trivia to get in your way.

The point about the Architectural Plan is that this is the plan from which you and your SUPREME Team will work to implement your Post-Traumatic Success dream. Of course the one thing we all know about plans is that they become out of date as soon as they're written! All the more reason not to get bogged down in the minutiae of the documentation method. Whatever you use will be just perfect for a first plan; you can grow into newer, better, more sophisticated planning tools once you've gotten started. Remember, taking the first step is the hardest, and we don't want to delay or jeopardize that by being scuppered by technology.

The Architectural Plan needs to have enough information in it to enable us to make a start, without paralyzing us with too much detail. You can always add to it as new information or ideas come to light. Ideally the Plan should include areas such as:

- A description of the target audience (if it's a business, a charity or enterprise that will involve communicating with others) to keep him/her/them front of mind as you plan the rest

- The overall goal in as much detail as is necessary to save you having to look elsewhere

- Tools and resources needed for your Post-Traumatic Success

- Criteria for success – how will you know when it's successful?

- Any dependencies – for example, if you're creating a website, what needs to happen before you can start creating?

  ☐ choose and register a domain name

  ☐ buy hosting

  ☐ ensure you have your logo in the necessary format

  ☐ content to populate pages

  ☐ link to email so you can capture email addresses

  ☐ products or services to sell

  ☐ a clear call to action for your audience

- Specific tasks to be carried out and ticked off

- Milestones or deadlines along the way

- The easy first step

The Architectural Plan is what will keep you on track when you find yourself being distracted by things that are not helpful or relevant to your Post-Traumatic Success journey. It acts as collateral that allows you to explain your Post-Traumatic Success to someone else; it is a tangible manifestation of all the information, ideas, thoughts, fears, musings, hopes, dreams, details and aspirations you may have been carrying around in your head for weeks, months or even years. It's the place where all these things can finally come out and become real, thereby allowing the storage space in your head to draw breath, heave a sigh of relief, and get on with the business of creating new ideas and dreams. In my experience, this is definitely easier to achieve with a mind map than a spreadsheet.

It's now time to take that easy first step on the route to creating your Post-Traumatic Success dream. Will you be making that all-important first phone call, carrying out web research for your niche market, buying a map of Australia to plan your trip of a lifetime or calling five business friends to canvas their opinion on the need for a new specialist charity? Whatever your first step, enjoy the moment and don't forget to celebrate your first successful milestone when you've achieved it.

CHAPTER 8

"We judge ourselves by our intentions;
the world judges us by our actions."
J. Dean

Enjoy the Ride: Top Tips for Your Post-Traumatic Success

I've thoroughly enjoyed writing this book and leading you through a process for creating the Post-Traumatic Success of your dreams! I hope you've enjoyed reading it so far. It has been an interesting process in itself, remembering the thoughts, feelings and emotions that were true for me at the time, rather than the cleansed, sanitized and rationalized ones that tend to live with me today.

Whenever you learn something to a level where you are quite proficient and confident, it can be difficult to remember a time when you didn't know it. Chip & Dan Heath refer to this as 'the curse of knowledge'. It can be a curse if you're trying to teach someone else that thing, and you have difficulty understanding why they're not getting it; teaching your kids to tie their shoelaces, for example, or helping them with their irregular French verbs. My own children aren't old enough to learn to drive yet, but I'm sure when that day arrives I will empathize with my mum's suffering as I kangarooed her car down the street for the umpteenth time, or stalled on one of the hundreds of hill starts she made me practice!

I have had to dig deep on occasion while writing this book, to really transport myself back to the time, back to the rawness of the emotions, in order to best serve you as you embark on your Post-Traumatic Success journey. If you've read the book from page 1, I'm immensely proud to be able to accompany you on this path; if you've just turned to the top tips chapter at the back, and you're still standing in the book store, I urge you to buy the book! You're not going to learn much by reading the top tips section on the subject!

The following are a few last thoughts to help you on your way, with my best wishes for your success and enjoyment.

Top Tip 1: Stretch the Pantie Elastic – Daily

If you take a new pair of panties (or anything with elastic) and stretch it once, when you let it go, the elastic goes back to its original shape and size. If you keep stretching it, eventually the elastic will remain stretched and will never return to its original shape.

When you start out on your Post-Traumatic Success journey, you will undoubtedly be doing lots of new things: speaking with people you haven't spoken with before, about things you haven't spoken about; learning new concepts and skills; trying out new

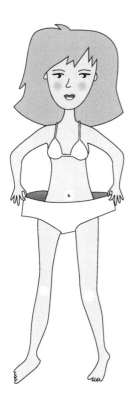

technology. Chances are, the first time you do any of those things, it will feel a bit strange – probably the second time, too. If you stop after the first 'stretch', the elastic which represents the stretch to your comfort zone will spring back to its original form, thus not retaining the stretch for next time.

Top Tip 2: Teach your Internal Voice to Play Nicely

It is a given that things will not go according to plan on your Post-Traumatic Success journey; you will screw up, things will go wrong, you will do or say things you subsequently wish you hadn't... and your internal voice will let you know about it! It will shout, call you names, play with your confidence, try to steal your self-esteem, and generally behave like the nasty child in the playground. If you allow it to, it will taunt you, make you feel small, sap your energy and your appetite for trying new things.

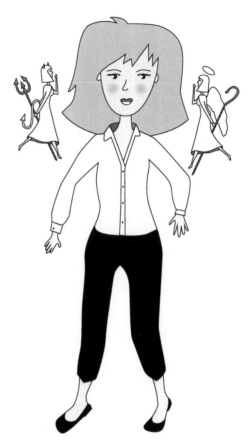

Here's the good news: the voice can be reprogramed, a bit like a voice on a tape, to say whatever you would like it to say. Why not teach it some nice words, compliments and terms of encouragement? It will speak whether you like it or not, so it might as well be saying something nice. As with Top Tip 1, it will go back to the default setting to start with because that is the habit. Once you are ready to break the habits of a lifetime, keep persevering, it will be worth the effort!

Top Tip 3: Choose to Live in Gratitude

Gratitude is such a powerful emotion, and plays a large part in all of the top tips. Count your blessings, constantly. And count again, just in case! I am a big fan of writing things down – start a Gratitude Diary and make a regular date with yourself to fill it in. You may need to think hard to find things at the start. Like everything, it will get easier the more you practice.

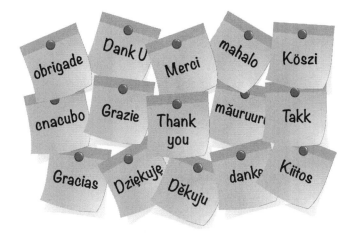

Top Tip 4: Choose a Resourceful State

Tony Robbins suggests that one thing we can really do for ourselves in order to get more resourceful is to ask ourselves better questions. Here are a few of my favorites (you choose the endings):

- What if I could...?

- How could it be possible that...?

- What would have to happen so...?

- What would I choose to do/be/have right now?

- What would X do in this situation?

- Who could help me now?

- What if I couldn't fail?

What resources could be available to you right now if only you were to ask yourself a better question?

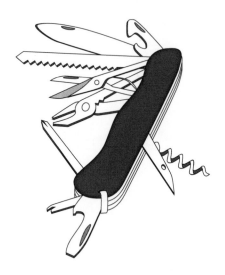

Top Tip 5: You are Enough

This is the note I would like to leave you with as you embark on your Post-Traumatic Success journey. You have survived a traumatic event in your life, you are still here, and still reading this book for a reason. Remember something I said at the beginning of this book: you are not your trauma. You are so much more than that, you deserve to be happy, successful and confident in yourself. You are most definitely enough.

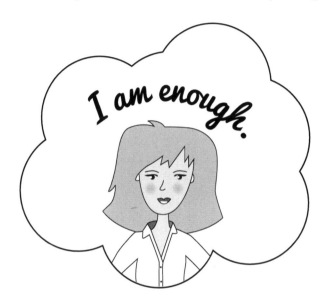

Proud to support
Breast Cancer Care

Diana Barden will donate 30p to Breast Cancer Care* from the sale of every book.

*Breast Cancer Care is a registered charity in England and Wales 1017658, and Scotland SCO38104. The donation will be made via Breast Cancer Trading Limited (CRN 2681072).

This book is based upon Diana's own views and experiences of breast cancer and does not reflect the views or opinions of Breast Cancer Care. Breast Cancer Care relies on the generosity of its supporters to provide its essential support services for free.

Visit our website at www.breastcancercare.org.uk

ABOUT THE AUTHOR

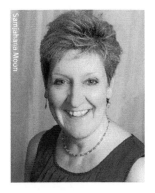

After obtaining a degree in modern languages, Diana spent 11 years living and working in Germany and Switzerland before returning to the UK in September 1993 to study for an MBA at Warwick Business School. She was diagnosed with breast cancer on New Year's Eve 1993 and against all the advice, continued studying full-time during her treatment, passing her degree with Distinction the following year.

Right from the start of her journey with cancer, Diana felt the experience gave her an opportunity to reach out to others going through similar traumatic events, and somehow help them to regain control over their lives (and bodies). As a volunteer peer supporter, helpliner and campaigner with Breast Cancer Care, she has helped many hundreds (perhaps thousands) of women come to accept what they cannot control, and recognize the choices they do have in how they live through their trauma.

Diana has spent the last 20 years delving into the hidden depths of the mind-body connection, the hard-wiring that determines how we respond and react to external events, and what can be possible when we start consciously choosing our own feelings and emotions. As a trainer, mentor and coach, Diana is committed to working with those who want to turn life's traumas into successes, and leave the world a better place as a result.

Diana lives with her two children near Cambridge, England where she runs Damsels in Success Cambridge, a movement for women who are seeking more success with ease in their lives.